BRAIN INJURY SURVIVOR'S GUIDE

Brain Injury Survivor's Guide
Welcome to Our World
All Rights Reserved.
Copyright © 2008 Larry Jameson
V1.0

Outskirts Press, Inc.
http://www.outskirtspress.com

ISBN: 978-1-4327-1620-2

PRINTED IN THE UNITED STATES OF AMERICA

Library of Congress Control Number: 2007939733

Welcome to Our World

"Looking Good and Feeling Strange" describes most brain injury victims because the large majority of brain injuries have no outward physical signs.

The Centers for Disease Control, a United States government agency, reports that over 5 million people in the United States have a long-term or lifelong need for help related to Traumatic Brain Injury. That does not include people who suffer brain injuries that result from strokes, or other causes.

More alarming than the large number of people suffering memory problems, cognitive problems, loss of job skills and behavioral problems is the fact that almost half the brain injury victims still have those problems a year after their injury.

This book is written specifically for brain injury patients, families of brain injury victims, co-workers of brain injury victims and anyone else who wants to know more about brain injury from a *patient's perspective*.

Beth Jameson is a Brain Injury Survivor. She has now lived for seventeen years as a brain injury victim and has developed numerous strategies for dealing with and overcoming brain-injury-related memory problems, cognitive problems and behavioral problems: the very areas of unmet needs stated by the CDC.

Traumatic Brain Injuries (TBI), the ones we hear about so much on news reports, are caused by external forces affecting the brain. Those external forces may or may not leave a visible sign. A stroke, on the other hand, is caused by internal forces affecting the brain. Cerebral Palsy and Multiple Sclerosis (MS) are brain injuries as well.

The CDC Fact Sheet also reports that a brain injured person's ability to manage stress, control his or her anger and control his or her emotional outbursts are among other unmet needs.

Each of these areas is addressed in this book with actual strategies that can be used by brain injury victims and family support members.

Patients and families living with brain injury must deal with the consequences of brain injury in a similar manner regardless of what caused the actual injury.

Larry Jameson provides information to the group of people he likes to call **the forgotten ones**: family and friends who make up the vital support network that will enable a brain injury victim to achieve a successful life. Brain injury affects family members as much as it affects the one who is injured.

We are going to show you how to live successfully with an injured brain. We are not going to give you any false hopes of returning to the *way you once were*; we are going to show you how to maximize your *new* brain and your *new* lifestyle.

We are going to teach you some strategies that will compensate for your injured brain in areas where it is having trouble: cognitive skills, memory skills and, even, controlling behavior.

Welcome to Our World.

Dedication

To the more-than one million people who suffer life-changing brain injuries each year in the United States and to the ever growing number throughout the world who find themselves waking up in a new world – our world. We further dedicate our writing to the millions of family members who become support personnel for brain injured patients.

A special dedication goes out to the thousands of soldiers victimized by traumatic brain injury while serving in Iraq and other areas of the world; men and women who have chosen to risk their lives for a more peaceful world.

Table of Contents

Chapter 1

Code Blue!!!

"Larry, you need to come to the hospital. There's been a code blue..."

"I don't expect her to survive..."

"We may need to amputate..."

"Larry, you need to come to the hospital. There's been a Code Blue. We're in Medical ICU on the sixth floor." Beth's mother, Mary Jo, sounded frantic.

I glanced to my left as I stepped from the hospital elevator and saw Beth's parents and one of her friends sitting in the family room. My heart froze, and I seemed to move in slow motion toward them. My father had been a funeral director and I was very familiar with hospital family rooms. A doctor I'd never seen before stepped from the room and walked toward me.

"I don't expect her to survive the trauma."

"What happens in the next 24 hours is critical."

Thoughts careened and ricocheted through my brain faster than those little spheres in a pinball machine. Before I could form a sentence, another light would flash inside my head and another bell would ring. What in the world was happening?

Two hours earlier I had been sitting at Beth's bedside talking to her about things at home and the surgical recovery process. She was excited that one of her co-workers, Lisa, would arrive soon with frozen yogurt, one of her favorite treats.

Lisa sat in the family room clutching a soggy, brown paper sack. The look of concern on her face told me as much as the doctor whose words were not really registering.

"A R D S."

"One of the leading causes of death in Vietnam."

Shortly after I had left for home so I could be there when our 13-year old returned from his fishing trip with one of my co-workers, Beth was discovered near death by a nurse. She wasn't breathing. Emergency procedures were quickly initiated. The surgeon's office was called. He was on the golf course. Time passed. A pulmonary specialist was called.

Time passed. Too much time. The doctor who met me getting off the elevator was the pulmonary specialist. Beth's mother was there and overheard the specialist berating the staff for not contacting her earlier.

A day later I heard the same 24-hour message with a twist. Beth's kidneys had stopped functioning, and a nephrologist was called in for consultation. Beth was sedated with morphine in the hope that her body would heal itself.

During this time, loved ones were allowed to see Beth four times a day for fifteen minutes, and only two family members at a time were allowed into MICU. Between my five to eight minute sessions I tried to work and to provide comfort to our children.

"We may need to amputate her toes," was the message of the day. Oxygen being pumped into Beth was not circulating throughout her body. The team of doctors was growing.

For the past year Beth and I had taken dance lessons. Dancing had become our primary recreational activity. There had to be an alternative to amputation. A nurse explained how I should massage the toes and feet with a *miracle* ointment. She cautioned, "Be sure not to get it on your skin. It could cause severe headaches."

I'm quite sure my glare spoke more than I would verbally express at the time. Me having a headache or Beth having amputations? I know the nurse was trying to protect me; my heart thought she was ridiculous.

The subclavian allowed the staff to hook several IV bags to Beth. Her kidneys were not processing the liquid, and her body was blowing up like a balloon. She gained 25 pounds lying there. Each time I completed my short MICU visit by getting on the elevator, going into the parking lot, and crying almost uncontrollably.

There was another family living in the waiting room with whom we developed a relationship. Their loved one was also battling ARDS. The time between those short visits to see our loved ones were spent nourishing and encouraging one another. A twofold sadness enveloped our entire family when their loved one died.

Not only were we saddened by our new friends' loss, but we were saddened by the sobering fact that she had died fighting the same problem Beth was struggling to overcome. Her body fought those many complications for fourteen days and, almost miraculously, she began breathing on her on. The breathing tubes were removed.

Mary Jo stayed with Beth when she was moved to a private room for another week. She asked her mom what had happened. Beth had no memory of the month of August.

Months passed after she was released from the hospital before we discovered that Beth had suffered an anoxic stroke in the hospital that resulted in a brain injury.

Her questions, however, provided guidance for Mary Jo. She discovered that Beth did not know she was married. She did not know she had two children. She did not know where she lived. More memory problems would surface.

Beth had forgotten how to clean house or cook. She struggled for words when she spoke. She had no idea what three times three yielded. She had vision problems. She could not remember what happened two minutes previously. She did, however, remember Buffy our Cocker Spaniel!

Beth had determination. She wanted to cook for this family to whom she was beginning to adjust. I took three cans from the cabinet, three bowls, a can opener and showed her how to turn on the microwave. I walked out of the kitchen apprehensive but hopeful.

Sean, our youngest, and I watched TV while Beth busied herself cooking her first meal since returning home from the hospital. Within minutes she announced dinner was ready with a qualification.

"It doesn't look like very much."

I went to the kitchen. There was a bowl of warm green beans. There were also two unopened cans and two empty bowls. She had forgotten that I had placed three items for her to prepare.

Her concentration on preparing the beans caused her to focus both her brain and her eyesight on the beans. We would later learn that she had no peripheral vision; she could not see the other cans or bowls.

Does any of this sound familiar to you? We're sure you are experiencing very similar problems in your life. It's very possible that you, like Beth, have no outward signs of what is going on inside your head.

You look normal so people expect you to be normal. If you had a piece of shrapnel sticking out through your skin, people would be a little more understanding. But you don't, do you?

That's why we're writing this Survivor's Guide for you. The medical community can provide you with statistics. They can tell you "things" you should do if you are experiencing "such and such". They can tell you how the brain is supposed to operate and about left brain and right brain issues. However, if your medical professional or medical team has not personally had a brain injury, they don't really know what's going on inside your head and your life.

It is, after all, that same medical community who today defines what happened to Beth as a "mild" head injury. Their definition of a mild head injury is far different from yours and mine. A bump on the head is a mild head injury; loss of peripheral vision, loss of motor skills, loss of mental skills: does that sound mild to you?

When we began writing this book Beth insisted that the words, *"Knowledge is power to a brain injured person,"* be included. Those words were inspirational to her because she knew that learning how to live with her new limitations would lead to a more productive and enjoyable lifestyle.

Knowledge about brain injury and how it affects individuals differently makes it very difficult for medical professionals to completely understand its wide-ranging effects.

We were given a pamphlet written exclusively for people who had suffered a brain injury and who were experiencing the new world of cognitive difficulty. The pamphlet explained diffuse damage and how coup, contracoup, and centrifuglar movement of the brain inside the skull caused that damage.

Tell us again who this was written for. Exclusively for a brain injured patient? Exclusively for a person who has cognitive difficulties? Exclusively for a person with a short attention span and who has difficulty with words? Let us tell you a bit about a brain injured patient.

Beth's boss visited her shortly before she was discharged from the hospital. He commented about how many *Get Well* cards she had received. She responded, "Yes, but I can't read them." It was to this brain injured person that a pamphlet was written which explained the coup, contracoup and centrifuglar movement of the brain that results in cognitive dysfunction!

Can you imagine what kinds of thoughts and concerns must have been going through the boss's mind? He and Beth had worked together for seven years in what began as a three-person office. Learning that she was unable to read the cards hit him as a caring person, and then it hit him as a boss.

So why has it taken us seventeen years to write this? Admittedly, we were finally prompted to action by the Traumatic Brain Injuries being suffered by our soldiers in Iraq. We know firsthand the new life they and their families are entering. We know the best information about dealing with this new lifestyle comes from those who have been there. We know that knowledge is power to a brain injured patient.

But there is another reason it has taken seventeen years. Beth has problems today related to her experience and her brain injury. These memory problems are of a different kind. She does remember events in the hospital. She does remember the breathing tube, feeding tube, the four IVs and the catheter. She does remember being tied down with restraints.

When we pulled her medical records along with everything we had written and all communications we had received from so many sources to review for writing this book, Beth could not hold back the tears as she read them. All blame for the delay cannot be laid at Beth's feet. I began writing her story numerous times, each time becoming emotional and abandoning it.

We welcome you to our world even though you'd much rather be somewhere else. Who wouldn't? It's a world where virtually no one will understand what has happened to you, and that includes quite a large segment of the medical community.

It is a world in which family members and friends must provide knowledgeable support. It is a world that offers very little support for family members, the very people who are so important to the recovery, retraining and re-emergence of a brain injured person.

The purpose of this book is to address the needs of both patient and family. We have developed numerous strategies over the years that we will share with you and actually show you how to use them, when to use them and why you should use them.

A few of your brain functions are inside a cocoon; our goal is to guide you in helping those functions break through that shell and emerge as a beautiful butterfly.

Again, welcome to our world.

Chapter Two

Beth's Message to Brain Injury Victims

"Your brain is unique. Your brain injury is unique."

"Brain injury is the leading cause of death and disability worldwide."

"Our world is different from that of 'normal' people."

"I was confused. Why was I having trouble reading?"

*"A **good** mother could help her child with his homework."*

"Never give up."

A brain injury affects different people in different ways. Each of us has a brain that weighs about three pounds, has billions of cells and millions of "wires" connecting the different parts.

What goes on inside the brain is shaped, in large part, by our individual lifestyles. No two people have the same memories, even if they witnessed the same event at the same time. How each of us perceives the things happening in our individual world is different from another person's perception.

Your brain is unique. Your brain injury is unique. Yet, there are common problems we all share that come from our brain injuries.

It does not matter how your brain was injured. You could be the victim of an IED planted near a roadside in Iraq. You could be the victim of a car crash. You could be the victim of falling down and hitting your head…or just having your head shaken forcefully.

Or, like me, you could have gone for a period of time without oxygen causing a portion of those cells and wires to begin misfiring resulting in an anoxic stroke. Most strokes result in some sort of brain injury.

Each year in the United States over one million people are treated for head-related injuries. Worldwide, brain injury is the leading cause of death and disability according to the International Brain Injury Association. An additional million plus brain injury patients receive hospital treatment in Europe each year.

We are not alone. Millions of people worldwide live in our world. Millions more family members join us each year.

Our world is different from that of "normal" people. Get used to it. A brain injured person is no longer normal according to society's standards.

Let me throw out a word you need to understand: denial. You will encounter a lot of people who will deny the existence of your brain injury. You may even be one of those people. Listen to me; it's okay to have a brain injury. It does not make you less of a person. In fact, it will make you a person who faces life's challenges and develops strategies to deal with whatever situation arises.

Most of the denials you will encounter are very good-natured and come with the best intentions. You will be in a situation where you will not remember some simple thing. Your brain is working a little slower than *normal* and you stand there bordering on confusion, frustration and, perhaps, a little panic.

Someone will say, "That happens to me *all the time.*" Who hasn't said, *"It's right on the tip of my tongue?"* Or, *"If you hadn't asked me, I could have told you."* Every person has moments of temporary forgetfulness.

To a brain injured person, it happens *all the time.* Please understand that *all the time* is not really every single time you talk or think; your well-meaning friend did not mean it literally, either. Trust us on this: your *all the time* is much more frequent than their *all the time.*

Larry and I have written this book as a guide to dealing with your new brain and your new lifestyle. It's been seventeen years since my brain injury and I still use many of the tools and strategies today that you will make a part of your life.

Welcome to our world. Sometimes it will be a world of mental fatigue, confusion, frustration, guilt and depression. It will be a world of paying closer attention, developing new habits and writing down your personal strategies. It is a world that Larry and I have shared for nearly two decades. He is writing a section especially for family members of a brain injured person. I must say that my family's support has helped me over many, many hurdles I have faced during the years.

Let your family help you, and never give up!

Not long after I came home from the hospital (and before I even knew that I had suffered a brain injury) I tried to help our youngest son with his homework. I was to read questions for him to answer. I looked at the page and became frantic: I could not read! How was I going to help him? He tried to make me feel better by saying it was his penmanship; it was then that I knew I had a serious problem.

I was **confused**. Why was I having trouble reading? I became **frustrated**. Have you ever stood in line waiting to be able to do something? And waited and waited and waited. Have you ever ordered a meal in a restaurant and waited and waited and waited for the food to arrive?

Imagine waiting and waiting and waiting for your brain to feed you some information. I know I learned those multiplication tables; where is the answer? Come on brain, help me out here. I know you know the answer. Give it to me. And you wait. And you wait. You get more and more frustrated by the moment. And then...

You feel **guilty**. A *good* mother could help her child with his homework. It is not necessary for the guilt to be based in truth; you *feel* guilty regardless.

Guilt leads to **depression**. I'm useless in my role as a wife and mother. I'm a drag on everyone around me. Is there a reason I should not just end it all right now? For some people, ending it all means divorce and leaving the family they cannot serve the way they once did. For others, suicide.

'I love you, Mom' from both boys drew me back from depression time and time again. Larry certainly did his part. So did my mom and dad, my brothers, my friends and my co-workers.

You need to understand the sequence: mental fatigue, confusion, frustration, guilt, depression. Learn how to recognize where you are. And, we are going to show you some ways to shift into reverse and back away from guilt and depression.

When I sense that I am getting frustrated at work and know I'm headed for depression on the Response Cycle, I stop and ask myself, *"how bad is this situation, really? After all, I'm not lying in a hospital bed. I can walk on my own and not feel exhausted with every step I take. I am free to look around and take in nature."*

I CAN TAKE A DEEP BREATH! For months after leaving the hospital, that was not possible. I remember how great it was when I first realized I could breathe deeply.

I finally say to myself, *"This is NOTHING; it is not a problem that cannot be fixed, and if there is no immediate fix, worrying about it will not make any difference."*

All of a sudden, I have a whole new perspective and then it's amazing how things generally work out. In addition to showing ways to step back from depression, we are going to show you some successful ways to deal with frustration and overcome confusion.

For starters, though, think **exercise** and **music**. Each can play a significant part in your new lifestyle.

Exercise, like walking on the treadmill, allowed me to get away from some of the stresses of life and lose myself for a while. It made it easy to take a step back from all the pressing issues I was dealing with and relax. It sort of renewed me to start again. I was introduced to exercise as part of my therapy when I was at the brain injury facility, Timber Ridge Ranch. Larry, being the great husband, bought a treadmill soon after I was released from the facility. Side note: if not for his love, encouragement and patience, I would not be where I am today. Whatever he thought might help me in any small way, he purchased or made happen in some way.

When I was trying to regain my productivity at work, he bought software for our home computer so I could sharpen my skills at home without the pressure I felt at the office.

Just as physical exercise helps me, I believe getting lost in **music** is a way to let the injured brain take a break from all the stress. It amazed me when I discovered that even when I could not come up with the next word I needed to use in a sentence, I could follow along with all the words in a song.

In my case, I guess that was because those lyrics were in my long-term memory which was not damaged.

At some point when I was in the MICU, I recall hearing music in my head and seeing everyone dancing to it which made me feel very happy. I know it was not real and I don't know if the medication I was administered made me imagine it, but it was one of the few times I felt happy while in the hospital.

Both exercise and music can play a vital role in helping you step back from mental fatigue, confusion, frustration, guilt and depression. Be sure to make both a part of your daily life.

Aerobic exercise such as fast walking, treadmill, exercise bicycle, running, and swimming get your heart pumping and moving oxygen through your body and your brain. Brain cells rely on oxygen to function, so give 'em a good supply.

Chapter Three

Larry's Message to Family Members

"The difference between the brain injured Beth and the 'normal' Beth is about like the difference between night and day."

"The grocery clerk told Beth the total was $20.00; she wrote a check for $200.00."

Welcome to your new and exciting world of living with brain injury. It is sometimes quite a humorous world as well. The humor part may come later in your world just like it did ours, but we now laugh about many of the things that have happened over the years because of Beth's brain injury.

In May of 1970 I married a beautiful young girl and began the journey as a husband for the first time. In August of 1990 I began living with a completely different person and began a second journey as a husband.

Beth, of course, is both of those people, and *they* are almost as different as night and day. As she has pointed out, brain injury affects different people in different ways but there are a few constants.

Regardless of how the brain injured person's personality was prior to the injury, you will, perhaps, find a new spirit of independence. Your brain injured loved ones desperately want (and need) to be able to make independent decisions and do those things for themselves the way they once did them. Right now they can certainly make independent decisions, but the decision-making process will be nothing like it once was.

In fact, it may very well never be the way it was before, but that does not, in any way, mean that your family member cannot return to a fruitful life of joy, productivity and making independent decisions.

Then again, you may find that your loved one is exactly the opposite. Rather than exerting a new independent spirit, they could easily recoil into a world of dependency. Either way, they will have a definite need for your help and support. Later you will find an entire chapter devoted to behavioral issues and how you can deal with them effectively. That chapter also examines behavior of family members: your thoughts and feelings.

One small portion of your support will come as praise. You should develop a habit of praising correct behavior. There will be more about this later in the book. Positive reinforcement is essential to helping your loved one along the road of becoming a successful brain injury survivor.

Beth wanted desperately to exert independence. You, like me, may have come very close to losing this person you love so much. You will develop a new spirit of protection. Do you see the beginning of a problem here?

You want to provide extra protection to a person who wants to assert a new independence, and those two actions are similar to mixing oil with water; they simply don't go together.

When Beth first came home from the hospital I sat in the floor at night watching her sleep. If she showed any signs of any kind of problem, I wanted to be there with her. More than once I decided she was not breathing the way she should be and shook her until I was satisfied she was okay.

Any time she was out of my sight, my heart pounded and I paced the floor. If she dropped a bottle of shampoo or a bar of soap in the shower, I rushed to her bathroom like a crazed wild man. Actually, I was a crazed wild man. Was I overprotective? Did it cause problems? Certainly!

My most vivid memory of our protection versus independence clash came one day when we were walking out of a mall into the parking lot. I stopped for a passing car but Beth did not see it and kept walking. I shoved my arm in front of her. Her head snapped my direction, and I could see the daggers in her eyes. It did not matter how good my intentions were at the time. She did not see me making a life-saving move; she saw me interfering with her independence.

On another occasion, *we* made a list of a few items needed from the grocery store. Beth drove to the store alone for the first time since her brain injury. I paced the floor while she was gone, thinking of everything that could go wrong.

The grocery clerk told Beth the total was an even twenty dollars. Beth wrote a check for $200.00. **Note:** if you write checks be sure to get the kind that makes an automatic copy. You do not want your brain injured person trying to remember the amount of the check so it can be written in a check register. You need to remember that they cannot remember! Fortunately for us, the clerk handed the check back to Beth and told her she'd written too many zeroes.

Today, you have the option of using a check card instead of writing checks. There is, however, a catch to using a check card: you must key in the pin number from memory. The very moment the clerk says to key in the pin number your brain injured family member will think of forty-eleven things, and not one of them will be that four-digit pin number.

We eventually obtained ATM/Debit cards. I accompanied Beth to the bank that first time for the purpose of setting up her pin number, and I wrote it down in my checkbook. A couple of weeks later Beth called and asked if I would get some money out of the bank for her. I mentioned there was an ATM machine in her office building.

"I know I'm keying in the right number. Did you change my number?" I could hear the anxiety in her voice, and I assured her that money would be waiting for her when she arrived home.

It will not be easy for you to let your loved one assert this new independence, but **it is vital that you do so**. You will need to provide assistance when needed. Your loved one will have already moved beyond confusion and frustration before asking for your assistance. He or she could very well be on the backside of guilt heading into depression. Help is needed to back away from depression. (There is an entire chapter devoted to Cycle of Response later in the book.)

Credit cards are another option at the grocery store. No check writing. No pin number. Recently, I've been asked to key in my zip code when using a credit card. Are you beginning to see why I do the grocery shopping?

Gift cards are another option, but they are an option I do not recommend. Imagine the grocery total exceeding the amount available on the gift card. Imagine all the decisions to be made at that moment. What needs to be taken out of the basket? A brain injured person does not need to be trying to perform math calculations under pressure.

Your support role as a family member will provide you with many opportunities to assist your loved one. Let's look at another new area.

You will hear things you have never heard before. The front part of the brain contains a filter not too unlike an air filter or water filter. Its purpose is to filter brain activities and emotions before they become words or actions. Please understand this is a very simplified explanation of a very complex process. Books have been written about what I just reduced to one sentence.

When the filter misfires you will truly hear what is on the mind of your loved one. Many times it will be the very first thing to fire in their brain and has no additional rationale added before being spoken.

Brain injury victim George Gosling, like Beth, spent two weeks in intensive care after a bicycle accident. As he began to return to the real world he discovered his sister standing nearby and talking to him. George said his first words were telling his sister to shut up and get him some #*&$@ water. *(See Sources of Information.)*

Christian mother and brain injury survivor of a terrible automobile accident, Courtney Larson, was sent to a nursing home because she did not have the physical strength to participate in rehabilitation. An elderly lady who lived in the home asked her why all the staff and patients were talking about Courtney. She told the lady that she had #"&$@ up. *(See Sources of Information.)*

Imagine sharing information with others without thinking about whether or not you *should* share it. Certainly we all vent frustration from time to time. That confusion and frustration consume a great part of the day for a brain injured person.

Beth once wrote:

"Shortly after learning I had suffered a brain injury, I was sent to a psychologist for cognitive testing. When the results were given to me, I shared them, in writing, with my boss.

I could think of no reason I should not give him the information. After all, he had taken a very active interest in working with the insurance company to get them to cover my treatment at Timber Ridge Ranch. I should have said *"no"* when he asked if he could include it in my personnel file.

I definitely would have thought it through more carefully had my brain been working properly at the time.

It's something I never would have agreed to if my filter had been working. I don't know if my filter is working better with all the time that has passed, or if my "brain" strategies have greatly overcome those early days, but I don't have this problem to the degree I had early in my injury."

The brain is an amazing organ. It controls everything in our lives, including life itself, with a precision that is virtually unimaginable – when it's functioning properly. Certainly it is still an amazing organ even when it's injured. That precision is not what it was prior to the injury, and thought processes sometimes produce unusual results.

Similar to hearing things you might not have heard before, you will see things you probably have never seen before. Living life to the fullest with a malfunctioning brain filter takes on a whole new meaning. You may very well see more of everything.

Your loved one may cry more often and about more things. He or she may laugh more often and about more things. Brain injured people have been known to become more flirtatious. Modesty may no longer be part of your loved one's personality. Think for a moment about all of *your* emotions – unfiltered.

You see a sad movie and your brain fires for you to cry. The brain's filter says 'it's only a movie' and the result is that you do not cry. Someone states a political or religious ideology that is totally at odds with your belief. Your brain fires for you to open up with both barrels about how wrong-headed they are. The brain's filter says 'that person has the right to believe like that' and you sit there knowing how stupid they are but not saying it.

You see an attractive member of the opposite sex and your brain fires go for it. The brain's filter says 'your spouse might not appreciate you doing that' and you don't go for it. Or, and this happens quite often, you do go for it and create additional problems for yourself. We have included more information about this subject on our website.

Perhaps you see a brochure or some promotion for a Caribbean cruise or vacation and your brain fires for you to pack your bags. The brain's filter says 'you can't afford that right now' and you make other plans.

Maybe you have always wanted to drive a sporty convertible with the wind blowing through your hair like you don't have a care in the world. Your brain fires go for it, and the brain's filter asks if you 'should really have a car that can only hold two people and that has no room for groceries?'

Now, let's remove the brain's filter from those examples above. I won't mention any names, but guess who drives a sporty little convertible with a vanity plate about a place we visit in the Caribbean for two weeks every year?

Before Beth's brain injury, we had never visited the Caribbean. Since then, we have been on four cruises and spent well over 100 nights on an island in the French West Indies. Did we come into a great deal of money?

The short answer to that question is the same as the long answer: no. We have made lifestyle adjustments. We cut back on many expense areas in order to visit Beth's favorite place on earth each year. It has certainly become one of my favorite places, too.

Living with a brain injured person will require adjustments in your life. Your loved one is still the same person, but is a different person as well. You must adjust to the new person, and you must reward them when they make progress. A pat on the back is good; words of praise are good. You need to add reward activities to the list of rewards. Beth and I had so many celebration meals that we had to begin a diet and fitness program.

Each and every day, several times a day, he or she goes through the mental fatigue - confusion – frustration – guilt – depression sequence. Each and every day, several times a day, his or her brain's filter will misfire.

You and I must show and speak our love. You and I must gently act as the brain's filter from time to time without being too much of a protectionist. We need to be seen as a helper, not an overlord.

Your loved one must know that you will provide whatever support *he or she wants*, not simply what you want to provide. There must be a communication among family members and the injured person that is open, honest and always available.

Do not be judgmental of their words or actions because those words or actions may be unfiltered brain activity.

Rather than responding to a request with a flat-out 'no,' offer an alternative for them to think about. If you don't have an alternative springing from your brain, simply say, "Well, that's something we can certainly think about."

Then, **think about it**. Do not dismiss it. Sure, if your loved one has a short term memory loss, the issue may be forgotten by tomorrow. In all probability, it may even be forgotten by later today! Your bringing it up at a later time for further discussion shows that you care about their thoughts, and it shows them that you truly want to communicate and provide assistance.

Add more humor to your life. Laugh with your loved one about something *they* did. Laugh with your loved one about something *you* did. Dr. Glen Johnson writes that a sense of humor seems to speed recovery.

I can't tell you how many times Beth has looked at me with a devilish smile and said, "And I thought I was the one with a brain injury."

Always available to you as a response to *anything* they say would be, "Is that filtered or unfiltered?"

There are some important tools we will discuss in more detail later, but you should make a few things a part of your everyday life: calendars, how-to lists, an organizer, more how-to lists, a computer with calendars, how-to lists and an organizer. Inability to get organized is common among brain injury victims.

You are more than a family member. You are much more than a loved one. You are now a support organization. You need to put on paper as much as you possibly can. Writing notes will help both you and your loved one track progress. The smallest forward steps are still *forward steps*.

I will be the last person on earth to tell you that it will be easy. You may believe in your heart, soul and mind that your love for your injured family member will sustain you through anything that arises. It will certainly help, but you should know and prepare yourself to see that love tested time and again.

You **will need** your own support organization. You need someone with whom you can talk and share both the joys and frustrations of your new lifestyle. There are many such organizations available to you, and we've listed several in the **Sources of Information** section.

Your best support will come from others walking in your shoes: family members of brain injured people. There are a lot of family members willing to help. There are a lot of family members who have already faced a situation that you are now facing. Find them, talk to them, write to them, and email them. Become part of a support network. We believe these people can provide some of the best guidance you will receive.

Write everything down. When your loved one visits a doctor, questions will be asked about how things have been going. What sort of symptoms is the patient experiencing? The doctor or nurse will ask a brain injured person the same questions they ask anyone else.

The *fly in the ointment*, of course, is that they are speaking to a different kind of brain. This one functions slower, may very well have severe memory problems and cannot provide comprehensive answers to those questions.

Beth still has regular visits with the "headache" doctor and still uses three types of headache medication and a nausea medication necessitated by the headache or medications for the headache. For each visit Beth takes a spreadsheet of headaches she has experienced since her last visit. On it she lists the date of the headache, the severity classification, and the medications taken.

Can you imagine trying to recall all the headaches you had during the past three months? How severe were they? What sort of medication did you take for each headache? Now imagine those questions being asked to a brain injured person?

Welcome to our world.

Chapter Four

Dealing with Doctors

"You can't teach what you don't know anymore than you can come from where you ain't been."

"A brain injury is not like a disease that can be treated with antibiotics."

"Beth was given no brain injury information when she was discharged from the hospital."

"You need a medical cheat sheet."

Dr. Joel Slayton was one of my "most admired" professors in college. One of Dr. Slayton's favorite sayings was, *"You can't teach what you don't know anymore than you can come from where you ain't been."*

The brain is one of the most studied and least understood parts of a human. Every brain injured person must deal with doctors and other members of the medical community **who have never experienced a brain injury.**

Their information, for the most part, is coming from a place where *they ain't been.*

One member of the medical community is your **Health Insurance Company.** While we are tempted to write many, many things about our insurance company we are working hard to filter our comments. We'll simply say we hired a lawyer who helped get Beth into a brain injury facility *fifteen months* after her injury!

The insurance company approved two weeks of treatment. Near the end of two weeks we would have a meeting and Beth's program manager would send a letter to the insurance company to get two more weeks approved.

Those seven-page letters always began, "Attached is the bi-weekly report which is a compilation of treatment information for each therapy discipline, for services rendered ..." Every two weeks.

After a period of time, part of Beth's treatment was to go home on Saturday and learn how to cook, clean house, wash dishes and clothes, etc. Then back to the facility on Sunday. Two days before Christmas, the insurance company announced that if Beth was able to go home one day a week, she was able to go home for good and that they would discontinue coverage if she left the facility again.

Who else is on your medical team? We will limit the discussion here to brain-related medical personnel. Very probably you have a team of others like Beth did. Are you seeing an occupational therapist? Perhaps you are in need of a speech therapist and a physical therapist. Do you have a social worker? Case manager? Proper treatment for brain injury requires numerous specialists.

Having such a professional, coordinated team is not always readily available to you. In many instances, family members must fill in the gaps. One of the purposes of this book is to prevent you from trying to teach what you don't know. We cannot teach you how to become a medical professional, but we can teach you how to provide support and guidance to your loved one.

It just might be your guidance that provides a breakthrough for your loved one. Here's a bit of our story.

Headaches are a common sign of brain injury. When Beth left the hospital she began having **migraine** headaches every six days.

Please remember she was given no brain injury information when she was discharged from the hospital. We did not know she had suffered a stroke while in the hospital. So Beth's life was six days of mental fatigue - confusion - frustration - guilt - depression followed by two days in bed with a migraine followed by six days of mental fatigue - confusion - frustration - guilt - depression followed by two days in bed with a migraine.

Week after week and month after month the cycle continued. Neurosurgeon One prescribed medications that had no positive effect, then changed the medications to others that had no positive effect.

I found Neurosurgeon Two who specialized in headaches. It was no easy task convincing a brain injured person to try out a new doctor, but Beth finally went along. It turned out to be the first positive step to a livable lifestyle.

Doctor Corbitt also performed those medication combination experiments to discover what was best for Beth and actually hit on a combination that reduced the number of migraines. We were thankful to have more than six days between those periods of darkness.

She was also the doctor who referred Beth to the psychologist who performed all those tests and decided that Beth should be admitted to a brain injury facility. As mentioned earlier, many months passed before that admittance actually happened.

Luckily for us, Arkansas was home to the **Timber Ridge Ranch,** and it was only 40 or so miles from where we lived. Our team of social workers, occupational and physical therapists was truly five star. There is more information about this great facility at the end of the book in the *Sources of Information* section. In fact, they have been very helpful in putting this book together.

When dealing with the medical community, you need to understand their limitations. A brain injury is not like a broken bone. A cast cannot be put on to hold it steady while it heals itself.

A brain injury is not like a disease that can be treated with antibiotics. Many brain injury symptoms will never go away. You compensate for them, and you succeed by doing what works best *for you*.

You cannot depend on a written prescription that will cure your symptoms. You should prepare to deal with doctors knowing that much of what happens will be trial-and-error while searching for trial-and-success.

It is important that you develop and maintain a good relationship with your **Primary Care Physician** (PCP). It does not matter whether or not you need referrals from your PCP to specialists for insurance purposes.

Make certain that your PCP receives information from your specialists. Your primary care physician will be able to monitor the varying medications prescribed by each of your other doctors and determine any potential problems.

It is also a good idea to develop and maintain a good relationship with your **pharmacist**. This will provide you with at least two members of the medical community monitoring all the medications prescribed for you.

As mentioned in the message to family members, it is essential that you write down everything about any medical conditions for which you will seek treatment.

Brain injury victims need a **medical cheat sheet** that is carried with them at all times. You cannot wear a bracelet that contains all the information you will need. Your cheat sheet will include information about your health insurance, a list of medications being taken, date and reason for any surgeries, childhood diseases and a synopsis of family medical history. You will find more information about this in *Little Ol' List Maker, You*.

Think about this for a moment. You go to the doctor's office and are greeted with the words, "We need you to update your information for our files." You are handed seven or so pages to read and complete. A brain injured person, with no help, will finish the paperwork next Tuesday.

One of the office workers may offer assistance by asking the questions and recording the answers. Without a medical cheat sheet, correct answers to the questions will be completed by next Monday.

Certainly the process can be speeded up even without a medical cheat sheet. "Have you ever had…?" *I don't know.* "Has any member of your family ever had…?" *I don't know.* "When was the last time you…?" *I can't remember.*

A brain injured person needs a **medical cheat sheet** that is carried at all times. A sample is included in the chapter *Little Ol' List Maker, You.*

Welcome to our world.

Chapter Five

Dealing with Your Brain

"No two brains are alike."

Meet Clinical Neuropsychologist Dr. Glen Johnson

"Think of your brain, for the moment, as being a small block of gelatin. Some of you may be saying you have been thinking that for quite some time now. We understand."

"Sexual activity can take several avenues of expression."

"The good news is that there are ways to compensate for your problems."

Your brain and the information it contains is not like any other person's brain. Sure, they all may look alike and they all may weigh about the same; they all have cells and "wires" and electrical impulses.

But no two brains have the same information stored inside. Your brain is injured. The problems you are experiencing are unique to you depending on the exact location of the injury.

Clinical Neuropsychologist Dr. Glen Johnson explains brain injury by comparing the brain to gelatin. Think of your brain, for the moment, as being a small block of gelatin. Some of you may be saying you have been thinking that for quite some time now. We understand.

However, now we want you to imagine running a knife about halfway through the gelatin block in two or three places. You step away from it and take a close look. What does the gelatin do?

Nothing! You cut it, or injured it, and yet it still looks the same. You may not even see where you made the cuts. But there is one other thing you need to do. Now, lift the gelatin upward.

Those cuts opened up, didn't they? You can see separation. Imagine millions of tiny wires running through the gelatin. When the gelatin was sliced, those little wires were cut. Looking at the separation, you can see how many of those wires may have been cut. It would not take a "slice" as used in this example. A tiny pin prick could do enough damage to change a lifestyle.

Tiny wires carrying electrical impulses connect areas of your brain that help you Think – Read - Talk – Organize - Understand – Remember – Perceive – Respond – Comprehend – Decide.

Those tiny wires connect parts of your brain that determine how you act or react in certain situations. Will you accept or deny? Are you optimistic or pessimistic? Are you comfortable with things going on around you, or are you irritated by them? Does a situation require you to speak calmly or shout? Do you remain calm or do you throw a temper tantrum?

A brain injured person, more often than not, will display self-centeredness. We could not help but chuckle when those t-shirts pronouncing "It's All About Me" hit the market. The whole world was practicing one of the primary behavioral issues of brain injury. We have an entire section of this book devoted to behavioral issues and how family members can help guide positive changes.

Some of those cut wires or injured brain cells can result in a person exhibiting extraordinary suspicion, increased depression, lack of motivation, and a general loss of control. Sexual activity can take several avenues of expression. Some brain injury victims report a loss of desire, which very probably equates to lack of self-esteem. On the other hand, and usually a more frequent response, is increased sexual activity and promiscuity.

These brain issues, in turn, may cause problems with family, co-workers, friends and strangers. You may sense that you look different because you feel different. You may very well sense that people can "see" your brain injury.

The good news is that there are ways to overcome or, at least, *compensate* for your problems. The other good news is that many of your early symptoms will simply go away as your brain reroutes information and retrains itself. Other problems are yours for life.

Even if you are experiencing a problem that will go away three years from now, you need to live with it *now*. You need to compensate for that loss for the next three years. In other words, you will learn strategies to make up for what your brain is failing to do.

During the early stages of your brain injury you will be feeding a lot of information to your brain, and some of what you feed it will be terrible, terrible stuff.

Beth wrote a letter than contained these comments:

"It's exactly 1 year since the day I went to the hospital. You would think that a person would **want** to forget.

"Why is it that I have all these memories of my time in ICU?

"I remember Larry being there and telling me to blow on some contraption to keep me from getting pneumonia. I hated it. I was so tired and didn't feel I could breathe very well. I just nodded in agreement."

You may have negative information from outside sources writing to your brain. For instance, before Beth received any information or training about dealing with her brain injury she received this letter.

"The Benefits Determination Committee met this morning and evaluated your request for treatment at the Timber Ridge Ranch.

"The Committee was unanimous in their decision that this is not a covered benefit under the Exclusions and Limitations that can be found in your Schedule of Benefits."

Not all negativity will come from the outside world. You will feed your brain quite a few negative thoughts simply due to things being different. *Why can't I remember that guy's name? Why am I having so much trouble reading? Why am I thinking so slowly?*

There was a time when you had trained your brain in so many areas that many things just happened automatically without you having to think about what to do.

For instance, you walk down the aisle of a grocery store and your brain remembers the brand you always buy so you walk directly to that item and it goes into your cart. Now, however, you stop and look at every similar item. You try to read, with difficulty, product information and make a decision, with difficulty, about which product to put in the basket.

A 30-minute trip to buy groceries can last several hours if you don't have a **grocery list** telling you what to buy. You will read more about this in *Little Ol' List Maker, You.*

The next page contains a cutaway photo of a brain and points out where some of the functioning occurs. Knowing where your brain is injured can help you understand more about your particular injury and potential compensatory strategies you must learn.

Of course, the interconnectivity of those millions of nerves running through your brain can affect several areas all at once.

Beth has no peripheral vision, which relates to the Occipital lobe. She also has problems making decisions, and that relates to the Frontal lobe. Her lack of short term memory is part of the Temporal lobe, while slowed processing of information is Parietal lobe stuff.

Our strategies for living with brain injury are laid out according to symptoms you are experiencing rather than where your actual injury occurred.

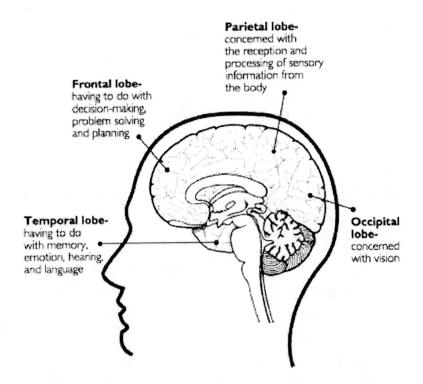

Parietal lobe- concerned with the reception and processing of sensory information from the body

Frontal lobe- having to do with decision-making, problem solving and planning

Temporal lobe- having to do with memory, emotion, hearing, and language

Occipital lobe- concerned with vision

Illustration Source: National Institutes of Health

More important than understanding the location of your injury and potential problems is understanding the **Cycle of Response** and the daily issues you will face.

Chapter Six

The Cycle of Response

"Your injured brain does have its limits."

Mental Fatigue

Confusion

Frustration

Guilt

Depression

You will respond to your brain injury. The injury will cause numerous changes in your life because your brain functions differently than it did before.

The medical community calls this the wheel of metacognition; we call it your **Cycle of Response.** *Metacognition* is defined as thinking about thinking. And the medical community certainly does a lot of that.

You, too, will think a lot about your new thinking processes. First, however, think about this. Imagine you have sprained your ankle. For several days, you will not walk normally. Nor will you walk as much as you did prior to the sprain. You do that for two primary reasons. One is because it hurts. The other is to rest your ankle while it heals.

It is not quite that easy to rest your brain because those little electrical firings are happening millions or billions of times each minute.

Your injured brain does have its limits. You will quickly recognize one of those limits as **mental fatigue.** There will be a time of day you will come to know as BEST THINKING TIME. For Beth, the morning hours are best because no demands were made on her brain while she slept. Those hours could easily be your best as well, and for the same reason. Just as your injured brain has its limits, you will quickly realize that your best thinking time has its limits as well.

The best thinking time for Beth lasts about five hours. Your particular best time may be shorter if your brain injury is more recent. It may be longer, but we would almost bet that it's not. A best thinking time that exceeds five hours would be rare for a "normal" person.

Once mental fatigue happens, you move away from your best thinking and, perhaps, subconsciously, you wonder why you cannot think as clearly as you did five minutes ago.

That "wonder why" thought leads to a time of **confusion**. You can recognize that you have entered your confusion time and back away from trying to absorb new information and decision making.

Or, you can plunder ahead with more and more questions about *why can't I do this? Why can't I do that? I did it an hour ago. I need to ask…what's his name…for more information. Why can't I remember his name? We had lunch together an hour ago.*

As more and more of these questions arise, you begin to reach a conclusion and move into the next stage: **frustration.**

Getting frustrated about not being able to do something you've done a thousand times is a natural response. Who doesn't get frustrated? A brain injured person, though, finds many more reasons for that frustration.

The source may be vision-related, word-related, math-related, memory-related or, it might spring from a lack of attention or be due to a lack of organization. Each of these is a common problem.

You begin writing some sort of communication to another person. You're about half finished when the phone rings, and you answer the phone. You go back to your writing. *Hmmmmm, what was I writing about? What was I going to say next? Oh, well, I'll finish it later.*

You lay the writing atop a pile of other unfinished writings. Just looking at the size of the stack frustrates you. A thought winds its way through your brain.

I can't do this. I'm not a good employee. I'm not as good of a husband as I was. I'm not as good a father as I was.

And you begin to feel **guilty** because you convince yourself that you are a lesser person.

You feel that you are letting down your family. You feel that you are letting down your employer. You feel that you are letting down your friends. Those **guilty feelings** will attack you with a vengeance.

Just remember that these thoughts are springing from an injured brain. It does not matter what part of your brain was injured, you will have these thoughts. It does not matter if you were involved in an automobile accident that was totally someone else's fault, you will have these thoughts.

Yes, you are a different person, but you are not a lesser person. Never give up! You will learn to do things for your brain instead of relying on your brain to do them for you. Likewise, you will learn strategies that will allow you to do things for your family members. Never give up!

When guilt is left unchecked, **Depression** creeps in. *My boss would be better off without me. My wife would be better off without me. My children would be better off without me. Everyone would be better off without me.*

These thoughts will happen. If you fail to recognize depression when it sneaks up on you, you will take action. Our social worker told us that about half of the marriages of brain injured people are dissolved. That is exactly the opposite of what a brain injured person needs. Family support is crucial to overcoming or compensating for the effects of brain injury.

This is one reason that both brain injury patients and family members need support organizations. Think with us for a moment.

Who are the people you most enjoy being around? Who are your pals? They are people with whom you share some sort of interest. That is the very reason **social networking on the Internet** has become such big business. Millions of people each day log on to share with others who have a common interest.

Most of us have numerous circles of friends. We like to dance, and we usually go to the same nightclub on a regular basis. There we meet with others who also like to dance and are regulars at the same club.

We also like boating. There is a sandbar on the Arkansas River known as The Hump. Each weekend dozens of boats gather at the sandbar, and a good time is had by all. We never see most of these people at any other time but, at the sandbar, we're all friends.

A brain injured person and a brain injured person's family members need to develop an additional circle of friends. Your common interest, of course, is the brain injury. Unlike dancing and boating, this new circle of friends comprise a wealth of information about dealing with your brain.

They are all familiar with memory problems. They are all familiar with cognitive difficulties. They are all familiar with social problems. Each of them deals with the rest of the world, and many of them have found strategies that can very easily benefit you, too.

There is probably no one more likely to tell you exactly like it is than another brain injured person. Whether you are in a group setting or exchanging email or forum posts, you can receive an in-your-face response that may be exactly what you need at the moment.

You are not the only person facing mental fatigue – confusion – frustration – guilt – depression. You are not the only person who needs to recognize where you are on the **Cycle of Response during any given moment** and take any necessary action.

Networking with other brain injured people or their family members allows you to share information, situations and concerns. That network can provide you with the exact information you need for a precise moment in time. We are very pleased to make this an important part of our website, braininjuryguide.org.

Welcome to our world.

Chapter Seven

Dealing with Getting Organized

"What do I do today?"

"My new best friend is a spiral binder."

"Getting ready to do something."

"Do you like salt in your coffee? Neither did Beth."

"What are non-thinking habits for most people become lists for brain injured people."

"What do I do today?" Brain injury victims from all over America, Beth included, stated that question was number one on their mind each morning.

While the rest of the world is singing their favorite catch phrase of being *proactive*, a brain injured person is the exact opposite. While others are trying to get ahead of the ball, the brain injured person is trying to determine what the ball is, where the ball is and perhaps, even, why the ball is.

A brain injured person, in the beginning, rarely has any self-motivation. Most of the hours each day finds them somewhere on the Response Cycle of mental fatigue, confusion, frustration, guilt and depression. None of those areas are conducive to self-motivation.

The **very first tools** you will need are **pencils and paper**. A spiral binder is best, and you will want one in a bright color. Why? It's easier to find. The lack of memory skills will cause that binder to get lost on a regular basis. It will just walk away...everyday.

Getting organized requires that everything have a designated resting place, and we came really close to abandoning this one. I cook while Beth's kitchen duties are loading and unloading the dishwasher. Well, that's how it once was. Technical difficulties (in Beth's brain) caused pots, pans, and dishes to walk away.

I spent more time hunting for cooking utensils than I did cooking. Beth was extremely diligent about unloading the dishwasher and putting things away. They were just not put in the same place twice.

After her brain injury we built a user-friendly kitchen so everything could be kept readily available. Some cabinet doors were made of glass so no one had to guess what was inside. Unfortunately, not all cabinets had glass doors and none of the drawers were made of glass.

More than once I would be walking around the kitchen, *"Eenie, meenie, minie mo. Can opener, can opener where did you go?"* That would be followed by, *"I love bread, and I love rolls. I would really love to find the bowls."*

You may find that humorous. It wasn't all that funny at the time. I now empty the dishwasher. And some of you are thinking that was Beth's plan all along!

Anyway, that's why you need a brightly colored notebook and lots and lots of pencils.

There is another reason. Remember that we said earlier that Beth had about five hours of *best thinking time*. When do you think those five hours begin ticking away?

Okay, you *normal* people think about this. You get up in the morning, have coffee or breakfast, bathe or shower, shave or apply makeup, douse on a sprinkle of cologne, aftershave, perfume, whatever, get dressed and head off to **begin** your day. Exactly how much thought did you put into each of those activities? Very little, we suppose, because most of them are habits and you perform them without thinking.

A brain injured person gets out of bed. He or she goes into the kitchen. It's brain time. Both cognitive and memory problems require that brain activity commence because decisions need to be made. *Do I want coffee or do I want a full breakfast? Well, I do want coffee. Where are the cups? I know I'm supposed to put something in the coffee to make it taste better. What is that?*

Are we overstating? Not one bit. One morning Beth mentioned that her coffee tasted "funny". I sipped it and discovered that she had *sweetened* it with salt.

Your notebook should have a section entitled **Morning**. It should include everything that needs to be done in the morning **and** it needs to include instructions for doing each of those things. Sample sheets for your notebook can be found at the end of this chapter.

How I like my coffee should be one item and it should contain the specifics. Now, it won't be too terribly long before repetition causes this to be a new old habit. Simple things like preparing a cup of coffee everyday will quickly become a habit. But that does not mean that every cup of coffee *will actually be prepared correctly.*

During times of mental fatigue and, especially, further down the **Cycle of Response**, there is no telling what might go into that coffee cup. Today, seventeen years after her brain injury, Beth forgets to add sweetener to her coffee. She doesn't add salt, though. Usually it happens when she becomes distracted while preparing it. With no short term memory, she cannot remember if she added sweetener or not.

Next, should I take a bath or a shower? What do you normal people do? You do the same thing you have always done. A brain injured person, though, may very well not know what was always done. They will stop to think about the choices. While it is second nature for most people, it becomes decision time for a brain injured person.

Makeup? You're kidding! While Beth was still in the hospital but out of MICU, she was able to have visitors. One day a crew from her office was scheduled to arrive around noon. Beth's mother laid the makeup bag on the bed and told Beth that she probably wanted to freshen up before her co-workers arrived. Beth looked at the bag, then at her mother and said, *"I don't know what to do with that."*

At the time, Mary Jo thought that Beth's memory problem was due to all the medication, sedatives, and the trauma, itself. Even the pulmonary specialist thought Beth's vision problem was due to the large amount of morphine she had been given. It wasn't until we actually met brain injury professionals that things began to click.

Beth's occupational therapist at Timber Ridge Ranch provided the much needed answer to the makeup problem. Write out a **step-by-step list of how to apply your makeup**. That list was taped beside the bathroom mirror for a couple of years...before it was moved to a drawer for future use, if needed.

Of course, if you've been reading since the beginning of the book, you know that Beth did not meet the occupational therapist until 15 or so months had passed since her brain was injured. Each day brought the intrigue of exactly how the makeup would be applied **and** if it would be applied in less than an hour. And I am being quite generous by saying *one hour*.

Today, seventeen years later, Beth needs about two hours lead time before we leave the house. Back then, we didn't leave the house very often. The simple act of *getting ready* that most of us take for granted would speed her through the **Cycle of Response**.

Remember, we are working with five hours of best thinking time. Some of that time was expended at breakfast. A sizable chunk of it was used getting ready.

Imagine a track meet where the starter yells, "To your mark...ready" (the clock starts counting for one of the runners)...then the gun fires. Even though the penalized runner may cross the finish line first, his time is slower and, thus, he does not *win* the race.

Brain injury causes things to be slower. Slower thinking, slower memory, slower decision-making, and, well, slower just about everything. That does not mean actions associated with those things are of lesser quality; it just takes a little longer to accomplish them.

Time spent thinking about anything cuts into the five hours of best thinking. **What are non-thinking habits for most people become lists for brain injured people.**

Okay, we've had breakfast. We're fresh showered, shaved or made up. A decision must be made about what to wear. This is difficult enough for a non-injured person. Throw in *difficulty making decisions*, and you can have quite a morning on your hands.

We converted a bedroom into a walk-in closet and organized the clothing. These jackets go with these pants and skirts. These blouses go with these jackets, pants and skirts, etc. Women's shoes – you're on your own!

Well, we did build a floor-to-ceiling shoe rack that has its contents rotated Easter and Labor Day. The shoe rack is on a wall across from shelves that hold the boxes of off-season shoes.

An essential key is doing whatever is within your power to move through the *getting ready* routine faster. We have found that being organized is crucial.

This section began with a brain injured person asking, "What do I do today?" Here we are several pages later and we have not even gotten to the *doing*. We've spent all this time getting ready to do.

Getting organized is prerequisite to getting things done. Imagine how difficult it would be to take a college course of Algebra II if you had never taken the Algebra I course. You could certainly do it, but it would be a lot easier if the prerequisite course was taken first.

Certainly things get done without organization. Just think of the United States government. We even have a phrase about the right hand not knowing what the left hand is doing. Our goal, however, is to do things easier and more efficiently. That's requires getting organized.

Welcome to our world.

Sample Sheets for Your Notebook

Morning:

Making Coffee

Use _____ brand coffee. The coffee can is kept <u>in</u> <u>the kitchen cabinet above the coffeemaker.</u>

Use one coffee filter. The filters are kept <u>beside the coffee</u> <u>in the kitchen cabinet</u>.

Open the top of the coffee maker and place the coffee filter in the filter basket.

Put three tablespoons of coffee inside the filter.

Fill the coffeepot with six cups of water. Pour the water in the coffeepot reservoir.

Close the top of the coffee maker, put the coffeepot in place on the heating element, and turn on the coffee maker.

Wait until the coffee stops dripping.

The coffee cups, sweetener and creamer are located <u>in</u> <u>the cabinet beside the coffee can.</u>

How I Like My Coffee:

I use ___ packet(s) _____ sweetener and ___ teaspoon of _____ creamer.

The blanks should contain amounts and actual brand names based on your personal preferences. There is a reason for listing specific brand names. Not all family members may use the same ingredients. You also might have additional cans of coffee that have various flavors such as hazelnut or raspberry chocolate.

Another reason for listing the brand names is that doing so provides you with a source of products when making a grocery list. More about making grocery lists can be found in the chapter entitled *Little Ol' List Maker, You.*

Does the brain injured person have a job, go to school or some other activity outside the home? If so, you will need another morning list: **What to Take When I Leave the House**.

One morning I called Beth, only to hear the cell phone ringing in the bedroom. So I called her office cell phone, only to hear it ringing in the kitchen.

Welcome to our world.

Chapter Eight

Dealing with Common Problems

"Common problems are those shared by nearly all brain injury victims."

"Word finding..."

"Math problems..."

"Although they were trying to comfort me, I wanted to yell at them, 'No, you don't understand..."

Common problems are those shared by nearly all brain injury victims. Each brain injured person must interact with other people, and most of those people have absolutely no clue when it comes to brain injury. That is not to say they do not have a stereotype of a brain injured person.

Cerebral Palsy and Multiple Sclerosis are forms of brain injury. Hollywood produced a couple of hit movies, *Rain Man* and *Sling Blade*, that helped people more fully form ideas about what a brain injured person is like. Karl, Billy Bob Thornton's character in Sling Blade, was mentally retarded, not brain injured.

Dustin Hoffman won an Oscar for his portrayal of Raymond Babbitt in *Rain Man*. Babbitt, of course, was an autistic savant, not brain injured. Most brain injured people would love to have the memory and math skills of a savant.

Brain injured people are not mentally retarded …well, unless they were mentally retarded prior to becoming brain injured. Yet, retardation is probably what most people think about when they think of brain injury. It is with some of these people you must interact.

Well-meaning Family and Friends

There will be a large number of family and friends who will treat you as though nothing has happened. This includes family members and close friends who simply do not have any knowledge about brain injury and how it affects you.

They are very well-meaning and fully believe they are interacting with you with the best intentions. Those best intentions, many times, will frustrate you to no end.

Word-finding is a common problem associated with brain injury. You wait for your brain to supply you with the correct word and you stand there looking confused. You will hear, *"That happens to me all the time."*

Math, especially multiplication because it relies so heavily on memory, is not as easy as it once was. We have already pointed out how Beth could not perform simply multiplication. You will hear, *"I have such a hard time remembering the multiplication tables."*

These are but two examples. You will run across many more instances of people trying to make you feel good by adopting whatever problem you are experiencing at the time.

Beth wrote out her thoughts about this one day.

This was so hard for me in the beginning. I "looked" normal? When I could not remember or find the right word, I would start to explain why I couldn't. Well, that always prompted the other person to say something like "oh, that always happens to me too". Although they were trying to comfort me, I wanted to yell at them.......... NO, YOU DON'T UNDERSTAND.......... YOU DON'T HAVE THIS HAPPEN TO YOU ALL THE TIME!!! You are normal, I am not.

There is another group of people who will cross your path: religionists. To them, everything will be okay if you just follow whatever their particular brand of religion teaches. Karl Marx once wrote that *"religion is the opium of the people."* There will be a lot of these people acting like they've had a generous dose of opium immediately before talking to you.

Attending church quickly became a problem for us. Beth's attention span was no longer than ten minutes. During those ten minutes, her brain was processing incoming information more slowly than it was coming from the teacher or preacher. She had no short-term memory. A few minutes into a class or sermon she would become more and more frustrated. That's stage three on the five-stage **Cycle of Response**.

You are in church. You are supposed to be in an attitude of worship. Instead, you are frustrated. Can you think of any place on earth where you would more quickly make the leap to **guilt** than in a church? Attending church became a great source of mental fatigue, and Beth got more and more depressed each time. We stopped attending organized church activities.

We certainly are not advocating that you not attend church. Far from it. You can find great comfort in the Book that guides your particular beliefs. At the time we made our decision, we did not know that Beth had suffered a brain injury. We did not know what was going on inside her head. We had not yet learned any compensatory strategies. We did not even know what a compensatory strategy was. We could not tell people what had happened to Beth because we did not know it ourselves.

Mental Fatigue

Mental fatigue can appear at any time. A contributing factor can be a lack of sleep. Another contributing factor can be a lack of exercise. You must let your brain take a vacation and recharge. One of Beth's strategies is actually a good example here.

She listens to music to help her brain escape. A small MP3 player holds more than enough music and about a 12-hour charge. The 12-hour charge means that the player must be taken *out of service* and recharged. So must your brain be taken out of service and recharged.

Set targets when you organize your day. Plan to do something for two hours. Your target is walking away from it after two hours. Literally. Take a walk. Relax. In the movie, *A Civil Action*, Robert Duvall played an attorney who went down to the basement for lunch. He had a radio there with which he could listen to a baseball game. He was interrupted by a young office worker who felt he had to work during lunch because there was just so much to do.

Duvall's character instructed the young man that he needed to take time each day for himself, find a place he could go to be alone with himself, a place where no one would dare interrupt him. Follow that advice.

You and your brain need some alone time where neither one of you interrupts the other. Let your brain relax. Feed it some music. Feed it some pleasant scenery. We don't recommend crossword puzzles at this time. No card games with co-workers. Sit out in the sun, close your eyes and imagine you're in a hammock between two palm trees on a beach. The breeze coming off the ocean is gently rocking you back and forth. No, you cannot have a Rum Punch to more fully complete the fantasy.

Examples of Setting Targets

Shortly after your brain injury, targets should be set for virtually everything. You see, setting targets will get you started, and many of those targets will become habits. You will need to set targets for home activities and work activities. By following your targets you will reduce mental stress and fatigue.

Set a target for the amount of time you spend in the shower or bath. Be sure to have a clock within view of the tub. A brain injured person has suffered trauma;

life has changed. There are so many difficult things to be faced that it is very, very easy to spend "too much" time doing pleasurable things.

Imagine you have only one hour to get ready for an appointment or to leave for work. That wonderfully relaxing shower or bath takes you on a pleasant journey away from the brain injury world. It takes you to a place in your mind where everything feels right and wonderful. You look at the clock and discover you have been in relaxation mode for forty minutes. Now you have only twenty minutes to finish getting ready, and here come stress, confusion and frustration.

You made lemonade out of lemons and, then, you turned them right back into lemons!

Set a target for the amount of time spent deciding what clothes to wear. Actually this would best be accomplished the night before but, since Beth could never do it that way, we are not going to insist that you do. She tried. She would pick out clothing the night before *according to her mood* the night before. Rarely, if ever, was her mood the same the next morning, and those clothes were all wrong!

This could easily be quite frustrating in the beginning because your decision-making skills are diminished. Those skills will improve a lot, and this will become much easier. With the assistance of Eric Clapton, I was able to provide a little early morning humor to help reduce Beth's decision-making stress. Clapton's song, *Wonderful Tonight*, had some very appropriate lyrics:

It's late in the evening,

she's wondering what clothes to wear.

I would be in my home office and see Beth go into the walk-in closet, so I would fire up Clapton as a reminder that she should not spend a lot of time choosing clothes. Well, for about a week! Then, Beth got fed up with it…but she got the message.

Set a target for the amount of time primping for work. This would include brushing your teeth, shaving or applying makeup, and doing your hair. There will be more about this in **Little Ol' List Maker, You.**

Why are we setting so many targets instead of, say, one target for getting ready in the morning? There are numerous reasons and about as many clichés. The longest journey begins with a single step, for instance. A person with information-processing and memory problems in addition to a short attention span does not need to be concentrating on a big project.

This is really no different than any competent planning. You know where you are. You know where you want to be. So, how do you get from here to there? You break the journey (project) into small steps. Accomplishing each step is considered a milestone. You focus your attention on each milestone victory and, before you know it, you've accomplished the project.

Set a target for how long you spend cleaning a room. House cleaning follows the *milestone rule* we discussed a moment ago, and for the same reasons. In the beginning a brain injured person will tire easily. Being physically tired contributes to mental fatigue and, by now, we all know that's the first step on the **Cycle of Response**. Again, **Little Ol' List Maker, You** will have more information about helping you set up a successful house cleaning program.

Without setting a target for each room, you could easily end up with one perfectly cleaned room in a seven-room house and six rooms that were never touched.

Family members who spoke of behaviors they had personally witnessed in a loved one seemed to all have one behavior very high on the list: the brain injured person never finished what they were asked to do. Making lists and setting targets will overcome that.

Set a target for time spent buying groceries. Of course, you know more about grocery shopping will be included in **Little Ol' List Maker, You.**

I used this one a lot. I could spend hours at the grocery store if I did not time myself. Actually, when Larry went with me and I was trying to decide which cereal to buy (for instance), he would tell me I had 5 seconds to make up my mind until we were moving on down the isle. I didn't like it, but I have to admit it helped me learn to push myself to make a decision quicker.

– Beth

Setting targets for your home activities will certainly help you get more accomplished. It will also reduce the amount of time you spend on those activities.

We do not believe we can overemphasize the importance of doing this. Perhaps the greatest benefit is that setting targets and having lists to help you along the way will make these activities become habits much more quickly.

Work activities have added pressure simply because your job is your source of income. There are very few people who can afford to be a stay-at-home mom or dad. Having a job can actually benefit a brain injured person because it forces the brain to work.

Students should also pay attention to this section because school is your work activity. While it is not your source of income, it is your source of future income. One of Beth's major problems was learning new things. Students, by the very nature of being a student, are learning new things every day. If that alone wasn't enough of a burden, each semester or trimester brings a new series of information to learn.

Memory Strategies

The first major resource tool you need is a **planner**. Unfortunately, we are not talking about someone to do your planning for you; we're talking about a real, organizing planner similar to those lining the shelves of office supply stores.

You can certainly create your own planner. We recommend that it be no smaller than 5 x 8 ½, and we prefer the regular paper size of 8 ½ by 11. The first page in your planner should be a one-month planning calendar. In other words, each day of the month should be listed with room for writing a note next to that date.

This page will be useful for recording medical appointments, haircuts, manicures, pedicures, beauty appointments, meetings, family functions, birthdays, etc.

Each day of the month should have a separate page. It should contain the hours for the date with room for writing a note next to the hours. Again, you would include everything from your monthly page that applies to the daily page.

More than that, however, is that you have a place to write down notes and thoughts. Perhaps you, like

Beth, have frequent headaches or must take regular medications. Record that information on this page. If you are taking medications, you will want to place a checkmark next to that entry after you have taken it.

I cannot begin to tell you how many phone calls I received from Beth asking me to check her pill box to see if she had taken her morning meds. If she had known to have such a planner, she could have simply flipped to that page and saved herself a few anxious moments.

One of our goals is to help people living with an injured brain and their family members reduce anxiety and stress.

The website, www.braininjuryguide.org, has blank *memory magic* pages you can download and print for your personal planner. Be sure to get computer printer paper with three holes already punched.

Sample Monthly Planning Calendar

	Month: July Year: 2008
Date	**This Column is for Recording Daily Info**
1	
2	
3	
4	Holiday
5	Vacation Day – Boating with LaDonna & Randy
6	
7	
8	
9	
10	Doctor's Appointment
11	
12	
13	
14	
15	Haircut
16	
17	
18	
19	
20	Lunch at Pedro's with Arden & Tony
21	
22	
23	
24	Counseling appointment with Joan
25	
26	
27	
28	

Sample Daily Planning Calendar

	Day: Thursday Date: July 10
Hour	**This Column is for Recording Daily Info**
6:00	Take Medicine
6:30	
7:00	
7:30	
8:00	
8:30	
9:00	
9:30	
10:00	Dr. Jekyll at Med Center
10:30	
11:00	
11:30	
12:00	
12:30	Lunch with Mike and Cristie
1:00	
1:30	
2:00	
2:30	
3:00	
3:30	
4:00	
4:30	
5:00	
5:30	
6:00	Dinner with Marilou and Bob
6:30	
7:00	
7:30	

It is important that your planner contain at least two more sections: driving directions and memory strategies. Each of those sections should contain a Table of Contents similar to the one below.

Driving Directions Table of Contents
Medical:
Dr. Tom Smith
Dr. Kelly Jones
Baptist Medical Center
Jenna Mabry, Physical Therapist
Support Group at Community Center
Personal:
Football Stadium
School
Baseball Field
Mexican Food
Al's Barbeque
Family:
Mom's House
Chad's House
Sean's House

The actual driving directions will be listed in the order you have written in the table of contents.

Driving Directions - **Dr. Tom Smith**
Phone: 555-1823
Arkansas Children's Hospital
800 Marshall Street, Little Rock
Turn RIGHT on Brookswood Road and go to Hwy 67/167 Service Road
Turn Right on Service Road and go to on ramp
Turn LEFT at on ramp to enter Highway 67/167
Stay in LEFT LANE and go past where 67/167 merges with I-30
Move to RIGHT LANE and go 3 miles to I-630
Take Exit 139 B onto I-630 and go 1.8 miles
Take Exit 2 B to Martin Luther King, Jr. Drive and go .2 mile
Turn LEFT onto Martin Luther King, Jr. Drive and go .1 mile
Turn RIGHT onto Maryland Drive and go .1 mile

Family members can provide great support in this area by helping prepare the driving directions. If Beth would be driving alone, we would go to the destination a day in advance to ease any concerns she might have.

A computer is very helpful in actually getting the driving directions, but it is always wise to actually drive to the destination using those directions to make certain they are correct.

Several Internet sites provide maps and driving directions you can copy from their site and print for your personal use.

It is also important that these directions be read, re-read and read again. Talk about them. Does your loved one have any questions or concerns?

Planning is essential, and a planner is an essential part of the overall program. Driving, at least in the beginning, should be limited to familiar areas with as little unplanned, impromptu driving as possible.

Another section of your planner is one of the most important items a brain injured person can have in their possession: **memory strategies**. It could easily be the largest section of the planner because it will contain actual how-to pages for performing numerous tasks. This section will incorporate many of the lists we have discussed earlier and others you will read about in *Little Ol' List Maker, You.*

While your planner will be the most important tool for making your life much simpler, you should plan to work closely with family members and other support groups to develop your memory.

Memory Seeds are small pieces of information that will grow into fully formed memory. One seed will be a family photo album. Remembering names is cited by most brain injury victims as one of their most difficult issues, and it is one that causes the most frustration.

Sitting down with a family member and looking through a photo album is one of the least stressful things you can do. You are not required to perform to any level of expectation. Your only responsibility is to look and listen.

You and your family support team will discover many more memory seeds that will help you succeed. Let's look at a few other ideas.

BRAIN

BRAIN is a memory strategy that makes use of an acronym that is pretty easy for a brain injured person to remember. Acronyms like *BRAIN* are used by just about everyone for nearly everything in our world of speed communication. *NASA*, of course, stands for the National Aeronautics and Space Administration. It also stands for the Natural Athlete Strength Association, the National Auto Sport Association, the North American Shippers Association and, even, the North American Saxophone Alliance.

FEMA is another acronym; the Federal Emergency Management Agency certainly has been in the news. Think Hurricane Katrina. In your numerous dealings with the medical community more than once you have come across *HIPAA*, the Health Insurance Portability and Accountability Act.

You have used acronyms and mnemonics since early childhood to help you remember things. Do you remember learning how to spell geography by using the mnemonic, George Edward's Old Grandpa Rode A Pig Home Yesterday? Perhaps you learned the planets with the sentence, My Very Educated Mother Just Served Us Nine Pizzas. Now that Pluto has been demoted and is no longer considered to be a planet, your very educated mother needs to come up with something else.

Acronyms do help us remember things. *BRAIN* stands for a series of memory strategies: **Be attentive, Repeat...Repeat...Repeat, Associate, Imagine, Never Give Up**. These exercises will work for anyone; we believe they are *essential* for people learning to live with an injured brain.

Be Attentive. This is probably the most difficult of all memory exercises for a brain injured person who is suffering slower cognitive skills and a diminished attention span. It is especially difficult when you are sitting in a group with numerous people speaking.

Being attentive is very similar to creating a word processing document using a computer. You record a few things and save it to the hard drive using a specific file name like *chocolate pie*. Hours, days, or weeks later, someone sends you their special recipe containing more information, and it is also titled *chocolate pie*. You save it to your computer's hard drive. A little screen pops up and asks if you want to overwrite the *chocolate pie* file already stored in memory. If you answer 'yes' you will replace your original information with that sent by the other person. The computer, of course, gives you the option of saving it with a new file name like *chocolate pie by Bob*. Then you have both pieces of information stored in memory.

Your brain's memory works a little differently. While two pieces of information about *chocolate pie* can be stored in your brain, the trick is getting the correct one back out of your brain at the appropriate time. You should know that volumes have been written and the medical community continually debates how short term memory, working memory and long term memory actually work. However, they *almost* agree that a "normal" person's working memory can process only one to four pieces of information before it begins "losing it."

Your desire is to learn (re-learn) how to function normally. It is your working memory that will be recording this information. Being attentive means you must focus on that piece of information. You must try to shut out other pieces of information while you concentrate on the item you wish to learn.

This is one reason we recommend writing down those things you really need to know. It is very difficult to shut out everything that will distract you because there are so many ways for information to enter your brain. There is a very good reason for the term, Five Senses. Vision, hearing, smelling, tasting and touching all send information to your brain.

Not too far from our house is an outdoor barbecue establishment that creates a wonderfully heavy aroma that permeates the air. It does not matter what we are talking about when we drive nearby, we always say something about that wonderful smell.

Be prepared for distractions. Know that someone will throw the switch and your train of thought will be interrupted. It will happen time and time again.

Your best be*ing attentive time* will very probably be right before you go to sleep and shortly after you wake up. Those are times when there are fewer distractions. Beth and I are exact opposites in this area. Nights are her best time for recording new information. I much prefer the quiet solitude of early morning. I wrote that sentence at 2:30 a.m., freshly rested from sleep and with morning's first cup of coffee close at hand.

Your day, and mine, consists of many more hours of cognitive processing than our *best time*. Information will be coming to you throughout the day during periods of high distraction levels. You can sooth that savage beast with music. It is a very interesting phenomenon how you can listen to music while concentrating and the music does not interrupt your thought processes. Music can actually help you be attentive.

Mental fatigue comes easily and quickly when you are trying to learn. During these times you must pay *close* attention to what you are doing. For some unknown reason, Beth developed a problem after her brain injury with the letters "b" and "p". She will think "b" as she writes down "p" or vice versa. Many of the notes she has recently handwritten to include in this book show those same errors – after seventeen years. She has learned to focus all of her attention on writing when someone else will be reading the final result. It would be difficult enough to explain a "typo" of b's and p's since those letters are far apart on a keyboard. It's even more difficult to explain the "typo" when it is handwritten.

Very rarely will handwritten information be made available to others. Bill Gates and Michael Dell probably never had a thought about brain injured people while working hard to make the world of computer technology available to each one of us. Yet, their personal computers and software products are of great benefit to the brain injured community. The Internet allows you to connect to hundreds of other brain injury survivors.

Shortly after head injury, a computer will not be at the top of your list of necessary tools. Memory problems are causing great confusion and consternation. Learning to be attentive and minimize distractions will be one of the first steps that must be taken toward a successful life as a brain injury survivor.

Think for a moment about the movie, *For Love of the Game,* in which Kevin Costner's character was a major league baseball player facing a career that was coming to an end. He would lean forward on the mound, and the movie emphasized that the crowd noise and all other distractions simply went away.

You and I both know that the distractions did not go away; his concentration on what he was about to do shut them out. That is being attentive, and it is that type of attention that will help you rebuild your memory at a faster pace. Paying attention to new information that you want to keep is the first memory exercise that helps lead you to the second.

Repeat...repeat...repeat. Being attentive brought information into your brain; repetition will help keep it there. You must perform what you want to learn over and over and over again – in the same way. Okay, so you have a memory problem! How do you remember how you did it so you can do it again the same way? Lists. Written instructions. Maintaining your planner. How many times will you read that in this book? Over and over and over again!

Many parts of life and the way we live day to day come from habits. Brain injury will cause many of those habits to disappear from memory. Remember how Beth put salt in her coffee, how she could not remember how to apply makeup and how she did not even remember being married or having children!

This is not unusual. Courtney Martin Larson tells of her brain injury this way, *"When I first awakened from the coma, I vaguely remembered Jerry, my daughter, mother, siblings...I accepted Jerry as my husband because he told me he was, but I didn't remember having a husband...I didn't remember much about Zachary as a person, much less as my son..."*

You will find more information about Courtney in *Sources of Information* and on our website.

Can you think of anything that should be more embedded in a person's brain than a spouse or children? Forgetting what to put in your coffee seems to pale next to that, doesn't it? How you like your coffee, however, is important, and it is a memory that must be added. You will very probably begin with a written list, but it will be repeating...repeating...repeating that will form a new habit of preparing your coffee.

And, it will happen quickly!

You will certainly use the Memory Strategy part of your planner to write down items you want or need to remember. You will look at this section of your planner every day, and you will read over and over again those memory items. And you'll reach that exciting day when you open the planner and quote that item **from memory** instead of reading it.

This really isn't a new concept for your life. You have been remembering "things" since you were born. Now, however, you brain needs a little help. It is not the sponge of a preschooler. Beth and I continue to watch in amazement as our grandson grows. It doesn't matter the amount of time that has passed since his last visit, he can walk straight to whatever he wants. Wouldn't it be nice if we could all use the *absorption technique*?

He doesn't just absorb new information; he also uses repeat...repeat...repeat. One of our computers is his favorite for playing games; the high-speed Internet cable and fast processor are right up his alley. He would give me directions, *"Papa, go to www dot ..."* Memorized web addresses come from visiting a site time and time again and causing that address to become a memory.

Being attentive to new information is the first step. Repeating over and over again what you want to know is step two. Step three is linking new information to your long-term memory.

Association is another memory exercise that can be quite beneficial for you. In other words, you associate something new with something old or something that is already embedded in your long-term memory. We mentioned earlier that we vacation once a year in the French West Indies. One night we were introduced to a couple who responded, "I believe we've met before." The gentleman looked at Beth, smiled and said, "Tequila, right?" And, yes, that proved to us and everyone at our table that night that we had certainly met before.

It really doesn't matter what you use for your association. You want your anchor to be something easily retrievable from your long term memory. You meet Bob at a baseball game; he becomes Baseball Bob in your memory exercise.

You go to a shopping mall and park your car. How are you going to find your car later? We recommend that you have a small notepad with you at all times for the purpose of recording information like this. What do you do if you forget your notepad? Find a landmark. Many parking lots have signs for Section A, Section B, and so on. As you walk toward the mall you keep repeating, "I will find D car, I will find D car, I will find D car." Well, assuming you parked in section D.

The next time you go to that same mall, park in the same section. And the time after that, and the time after that. Make your parking space a **habit**.

Okay, you parked in a lot that has no signs. Let's take a picture for your brain. From your car, look directly to the mall entrance and then look the opposite direction. What landmark do you see that is in a straight line from the mall entrance to your car? By the way, don't choose another car that might drive off while you're shopping. Make sure it's a real landmark like a building or a flag or a light pole.

Associating similar items, also called grouping, is another memory exercise. This is especially good for errands and shopping. Just yesterday Beth left the house to get her nails done, pick up medication and get wrapping paper for a gift. She developed a plan that would take her to the nail studio, then by the pharmacy, and then to a local store where she would pick up the last item. *Nail, pills and wrapping paper* was her association. For security she also carried a note that contained the three items. While getting her nails done, she was distracted and forgot she had the note. Instead of driving straight at the intersection that would take her to the pharmacy, she turned right and came home – without the pills and paper. *Seventeen years after her injury!*

Association is the first necessary step. Now you should really put those items in an order that allows you to first accomplish the items that offer the *least* distraction. Beth based her grouping on the safest driving route, and she certainly cannot be faulted for that. Safety is always at the top of our list when planning anything.

Memory exercises and strategies will work. They will help you more quickly adjust to your new life. It *is* a new life. Make no mistake about that. Let's look ahead.

Imagine the end result of your memory training. Imagine your future memory being much better than it is today. Imagine life with less confusion and frustration.

An injured brain is just that: an injured brain. You still have the ability to learn; you still have the ability to succeed at your chosen projects. And you can certainly make your memory work more efficiently. Will it work efficiently 100% of the time? No; and that puts you in a class with everyone else because no brain performs at 100% each and every day.

Using your imagination allows your brain to tell you a few things. Take a little time to listen. We are not going to delve into the left-brain and right-brain issues so eloquently and not-so-eloquently written about by those in the medical community.

Your particular brain injury may have triggered one side of your brain to become more dominant that it once was. Beth became quite good at drawing. She will be the first to tell you that prior to her brain injury, she had problems drawing stick figures. Afterward, she was quite skilled. She could virtually duplicate a photo.

She was able to draw a horse *from memory*! Her family had raised horses the first seventeen years of her life. She remembered them, and she could draw them. It was an amazing discovery about her new brain.

More importantly, she was using her brain and forcing it to provide information to her. A different kind of association appeared. She began associating activities she wanted to perform with long-term memories.

Use your imagination. Could you take photos and sell them? Could you write a magazine article or a book about your brain injury experience? Imagine. What can you do with your new brain?

Rather than running up the Cycle of Response because you cannot do some things you once did, think of what you can do now!

You knew this was coming: *make a list*. This will be a fun list because you should write down things you want to do and places you want to visit. *I want to earn an income working from home* is on the wish list of millions of people throughout the world.

Doing something positive, constructive, satisfying, fulfilling and income-producing from home is within the reach of most brain injured individuals. An injured brain continues to function. It continues to learn. It continues to create new memories. It continues to be productive. You can harness the power of the *new you*.

I mentioned earlier about being married to Beth Number One (before brain injury) and Beth Number Two (after brain injury). I have been fortunate to be married to *"two"* wonderful ladies. The second one has a more independent spirit and is far more willing to explore new ideas.

She doesn't hide her feelings, and that has opened up a whole new world of communication between us. Of course she tried for quite some time to become the way she once had been. She wanted to be Beth Number One, but she finally decided to improve Beth Number Two. That decision is probably one of the most important ones she made that has led to a successful lifestyle.

She began to imagine a better life with brain injury playing a minor part. Her brain is still injured; she still has those *"memory moments"* and she still has problems with her vision. But she no longer concentrates on the things that are not perfect.

Beth has imagined a new life, a new way of living. Use your imagination to dream about the future. Imagine what you want to do in that future. Write it down. Think about it everyday. Work to make it happen, and...

Never Give Up. Family members, this is an area where you can prove to be a great help or an even bigger hindrance. Family members tend to be the first ones to say, *"You can't do that."*

Think for a moment about the day when Jesus was teaching by the Sea of Galilee. Parable after parable came out of his mouth. He spoke some of the most significant words about how to live that have ever been spoken. Yet, what did some of the people do?

Who is this guy? Who does he think he is? Isn't he the carpenter's son? We know his mother Mary. We know his brothers James, Joses, Simon and Judas. His sisters still live here.

Matthew 13:57 says, *"And they were offended in him."*

The answer Jesus gave that day is as relevant today as it was then, *"A prophet is not without honor, save in his own country, and in his own house."*

Those who knew the *"old"* you will be among the first to say that the *"new"* you cannot achieve your goals. In 1977, I had the wonderful opportunity to stand on the *mount* beside the Sea of Galilee. Standing there made it quite easy to imagine the thousands of people gathered on that spot centuries earlier. Today, it is easy to imagine that some of them would be naysayers, proclaiming that someone they knew could not amount to much.

History has certainly proven the people of the first century were wrong about Jesus; the naysayers today are equally wrong when they say you cannot achieve those items on your list.

So you have an injured brain! Actually, you have a new brain, one that thinks, dreams and guides you along the paths you will journey in your *new* life. That's exactly what everyone else's brain does. For the moment, your brain is processing information a little slower, but it is still processing information.

Your new brain is having memory problems, but you have made a decision to retrain your memory. You have decided to use tools and strategies that will make your life more enjoyable and productive.

Never give up on your dreams. Never give up on becoming the person you want to become. Never give up on yourself.

Family members, the challenge posed at the start of this section is one that only you can meet. You can be the best cheerleader available, or you can be like those people questioning Jesus beside the Sea of Galilee. Call it fate or whatever, but you have been chosen for this role.

You do not have an easy task. It is no simple matter to be a cheerleader and, at the same time, not give false hope. Brain injury victims, like babies, don't come with a manual that shows you exactly what to do and when to do it.

Beth and I would love to say that everything you can do to help your family member is contained in this book. We cannot. As previously mentioned, each brain injury is specific to the individual person.

While most people who have suffered an injury to their brain can benefit from most of the information in this book, *most is not all*. In military terms, you serve as the forward observer. You are the one who will see what issues need to be addressed, and you will be the one who calls for whatever ammunition is needed.

Brain injury survival requires a team effort, and each team must have a coach. The doctors and therapists who are part of your team are like coaches sitting up in the press box during a football game. They have a view of the overall situation and can provide strategic advice, but you are the coach on the field witnessing the individual struggles. You see the action up close. We hope you will use this book as your playbook, and never give up.

Daily Strategies

While improved memory skills will provide a great long-term benefit to your new life, there are a great number of immediate issues, most of which are right in front of you day after day. Some issues may seem trivial. Trust us; they're not!

Do you watch television? Does your television have a remote control? Do you have a VCR or DVD or cable hookup? Do you also have a sound system hooked to your television? How many remote controls do you have for your entertainment system? You may need to do what Beth did.

Identify the remote control device that turns the television on and off. Apply a piece of colored adhesive tape to it. On the back of the unit Beth taped instructions to help her find the on/off button, volume control and how to change channels.

Those two simple items provided independence for watching television. Sure, she was dependent on the "helpers" but not on any other person. That is of utmost importance to a person wanting to be independent, or needing to develop more independence.

Do you cook? Microwave meals count as cooking so there is a very good chance you plan meals without ever getting near a hot stove. Beth's mother, Mary Jo, is a list maker supreme when it comes to Thanksgiving and the family gathering at her house. Her long list includes every item that she will prepare and a few preparation notes like "*Carol and Larry to peel potatoes*". It has become a family tradition for my father-in-law and me, and it renews my memory of military days on KP.

You will certainly need a list of items to be prepared, but you will also need information on that list about the actual steps to be taken during preparation. It is not good to forget to add water to that pot of boiling nothing! Nor will delicious mashed potatoes result from forgetting to put the expertly peeled potatoes in the boiling water. How long do they boil? Write it down.

Be careful here. Someone will tell you, "Let the potatoes boil until a fork easily slides through one of the pieces." Would that be five minutes or five hours from the start time? A cookbook or a hand full of recipes from

Aunt Sally can provide needed guidance about the actual cooking time.

On your list, you would write down the time you actually placed the potatoes in the boiling water as well as the time you should perform the *fork test*. You will be looking at your list during the entire meal preparation, and you will be crossing through items, or making large checkmarks, when they are completed.

The lack of a line drawn through mashed potatoes will remind you to look back at that part of your list. You will find a sample Meal Planning List and a sample Meal Preparation List in **Little Ol' List Maker, You**. You can download copies at our website, braininjuryguide.org.

Do you shop for groceries? Of course you know there is going to be a list involved when it comes to grocery shopping, but there are a few more things to consider. You do not take your grocery list and walk out the door.

Will you need car and house keys? Will you need a cell phone? Will you need a checkbook or credit card? Will you need a driver's license? You probably need your organizer with driving directions to the grocery store.

And you need a time limit. It is important for you to have a target time for leaving the grocery store.

Beth has already mentioned the need for having a *target* for grocery shopping and how much she used it. It will be equally important for you so you don't spend the morning or afternoon debating the value of potato chips.

Do you clean house? Cleaning house is similar to cooking because you need a list of things to do, items that will help you complete the *to do list* like mop, broom, vacuum cleaner and, very probably, instructions for using the vacuum cleaner.

Will you be dusting and polishing furniture? Your family support team will help prepare the list. The polish you use on wooden furniture is not the same polish you use on leather or vinyl furniture, nor is it the same polish you would use on a smooth top range.

How much soap goes in the dishwasher? How much liquid soap should you use if you wash dishes by hand? The television commercial says you only need a drop or two; what does your family support team say?

You will quickly see the value of the *Little Ol' List Maker, You* and the downloadable lists on our website simply by thinking of things you do each and every day. Or, things you should be doing every day!

Do you fly on commercial airlines? Last minute changes and quick decisions are not the strong suit of most people, and they are very far down the list of "things I want to do today" for a brain injured person.

International flights have a weight limit of 50 pounds per piece of luggage. On a recent flight, Beth and I arrived at the airport with one bag weighing 27 pounds and the other weighing 55. The lighter bag was Beth's and it had been meticulously packed in sections so she could easily find everything. We thought for a moment about shifting from one bag to the other and then paid the $25 for an overweight bag. We have revised our packing list for the next trip.

That, however, is just one item for your airline strategy list. Security is another, and it changes every few months. It is very important that you visit the airport website, the airline website and, possibly, the Homeland Security website for the latest information. We attempt to keep updated information on our website to provide a central source of information for you.

Another item you must consider is the actual walk through security.

The security agent in Los Angeles made it very clear, "You do not have to take your shoes off, but if you don't you will be spending some quality time with one of our agents." Plan the clothing you will wear as well as what will be in any pockets. Jackets must be removed and pockets must be emptied.

Compare the list of items you plan to pack to the *prohibited items list* published by the government. There are some items you can pack in luggage to be checked that you cannot pack in carry-on luggage. It is very, very important that you plan well in advance of your flight. And, understand this: it's confusing to everyone.

Of course you will need your government-issued photo identification and a ticket. Will you use electronic tickets? Do you know how to operate the machine with the pressure of people waiting behind you? Yes, the cheat sheet is in your planner, and your planner is right there in your carry-on luggage.

If that wasn't enough, let's talk about a major area of stress: **finding your gate**. This may appear to be quite a simple matter, but think about changing planes at one or more airports in route to your destination.

Along with your airport cheat sheet you should have maps of any airports at which you will change to another plane. Fortunately, airport websites have just such a map that you can print.

Your ticket reservation or itinerary will contain the gate information you need. Circle your arrival gate and your departure gate on the map. Visualize what you must do to get from one gate to another. The tumultuous atmosphere in most airports can easily bring on *The Mall Effect* that quickly can add confusion to your situation.

Find an airport employee and ask directions. If you are feeling really stressed out, tell that employee that you have a medical condition and need assistance getting to your gate. Enjoy riding the golf cart. More than that, enjoy your stress-free ride through the airport.

You should never feel embarrassed to ask for assistance. And that doesn't apply only to airports. We live in a world of merchandising, and that means grocery stores move products from shelf to shelf and aisle to aisle. You will find yourself going down Aisle C to buy a can of green beans and discover that Aisle C now has Baby Food.

Yes, there will be green beans on the Baby Food aisle but it's probably not exactly what you had in mind. Of course, if your goal is to give up cooking to another family member, serving baby food one meal just might do the trick.

Overload Strategies

Make the world go away is much more than lyrics to a song. Each of us has those days when it seems as if the world is resting squarely on our shoulders. *"How was your day?"* That question, or a variation of it, is asked probably more than, *"Mommy, where did I come from?"*

Now let's apply those very same stressful days to an injured brain. It's a brain processing information more slowly; it's a brain having difficulty remembering. It is a brain constantly moving up and down that old Cycle of Response: mental fatigue, confusion, frustration, guilt and depression.

Overload happens when there are more demands being made on your brain than it can handle at a given moment. It's also referred to as the *Mall Effect.* You go to a mall to pick up a pair of shoes and come home with a pair of pants and three new shirts.

Why do people do that? Why do they buy things they did not specifically go to purchase? Merchandisers spend a great deal of time trying to come up with ways to divert a shopper's brain. You don't think those people cooking and giving away free samples at the grocery store are doing so out of the goodness of their hearts, do you?

Shopping malls concentrate the efforts of dozens of merchandisers under one roof with the goal of brain overload that results in sales, sales and more sales. And it works exactly as planned.

Slower cognitive processing invites overload. You have probably heard a very popular phrase, *"That's more information than I need."* That is certainly true for a person with a brain injury. The Information Age has many good points. Some people think we have entered the *Too Much Information Age*.

A brain injured individual lives in the *Too Much Information Age* daily. One of the better ways to handle an overload situation is by using lists, using your planner, and setting time targets. If information coming at you is not planned in advance, simply say, *"No, thank you."*

It is not difficult saying, *"No, thank you,"* to that sweet lady at the grocery store offering you a 500-calorie bite of aromatic sausage. It is not easy saying it to your boss.

That's when you say, *"Hold on just a minute. Let me write this down so I make sure I do it exactly the way you want it."* That simple statement stopped the information dead in its tracks until you could better prepare for it. If you were not working in 21st Century Corporate America or England, or Canada or Germany or wherever, that might have impressed your boss that you would be so diligent to get the instructions or request exactly right.

For now, however, just be thankful that you have a little more time to respond. The simple act of writing that information will focus your thought processes where they need to be. It also gives you an opportunity to think about it and offer an appropriate response.

Depending on the difficulty of those instructions or request, you might need to buy more time by simply looking up with a smile and saying, *"My brain is fried today; can I get back with you on this tomorrow?"* Of course, you know your boss better than we do. You know what you can say and what you can do. You know how receptive he or she would be to that statement.

You will want to develop your personal *"overload deflection"* statements. None of us can avoid situations of potential overload, but we can develop strategies to help get past them.

Beth, on some days, will stay late at her office so she can have *"quiet time with her to do list"*. On other days, she's out of there without the least possibility of the door hitting her backside.

Spend some time with your brain and learn how it is working each and every day. Learn how to recognize when it's full. Pay attention to your breathing. Stress will cause a change in your breathing pattern. That change should be your overload signal.

Perhaps you feel apprehension creeping into your thoughts. That's another overload signal.

If at all possible, back away from the situation. Take a walk. Listen to music. Do something you want to do. Relax.

Chapter Nine

Dealing with Behavioral Issues

"The good news is that many of these negative behaviors will go away..."

"I've told you this a million times! Why can't you get it?"

"Keep it simple."

"Communicate freely."

"Praise proper behavior"

"Encourage independence."

Every brain injured person will have behavioral changes to some degree. It is very normal for them to not act "normal." They are going through periods of mental fatigue, confusion, frustration, guilt and depression.

You may quickly see mood changes and increased irritability. Who wouldn't be irritated with all these new things happening inside the brain? They have difficulty remembering people's names, places and, even, how to do many things that were so easily done in the past.

Irritation can quickly escalate to anger which will manifest itself as slamming a door or slamming an object down on a counter or the floor. It might manifest itself in hurtful words directed at anyone within earshot.

It is important, therefore, for both the brain injured person and family members to understand that behavioral issues will arise and that certain steps can be taken to deal responsibly with them.

The good news is that many of these negative behavioral changes will go away as the injured person moves from being a victim to becoming a survivor.

We live in a world in which behavior that is not considered "normal" is considered to be "bad behavior."

A brain injured person, for the most part, cannot control behavioral issues any better than they can control memory and cognitive issues. Each one presents its own challenge to be overcome with re-learning and training.

While well-meaning family and friends all have "forgetful memories" and are so willing to share that information with a person whose brain has been injured, behavior is different. You will never hear the words, *"Oh, I do that all the time,"* when a door is slammed in anger or profanity turns the air blue.

Behavior issues come from the front area of the brain where emotions are filtered...or not! Many times, inappropriate behavior is the result of cumulative actions that have occurred over a period of time throughout the day.

Remember the **Cycle of Response**: mental fatigue – confusion – frustration – guilt – depression. Behavioral issues erupt during the cycle because the person does not recognize the path they're traveling and they continue forward. Understanding the cycle and taking a "time out" to back away and rest the brain is essential to improved behavior.

Family members must recognize the road to improved behavior can be very long and filled with potholes. You, too, will be traveling through the **Cycle of Response**. There will be moments of sheer exasperation as you try to be supportive.

Society has adopted many colorful phrases to describe overload. *"That's the straw that broke the camel's back."* *"He reached his boiling point."* Family members will become quite familiar with that legendary straw. While you are observing your loved one for signs of confusion, frustration and depression, you must realize that you, too, will exhibit signs that you are reaching your boiling point.

Feeling mentally and emotionally drained is an early sign that you need some "me time." While your family member has very probably taken up residence with the *me generation* and is proudly wearing the "It's All About Me" t-shirt, you need your own t-shirt: "It's Kinda, Sorta About Me, Too."

Those very thoughts will make you feel guilty. How can you think about yourself when your loved one is going through so much stress and so many changes?

You are in good company, and lots of it, too. Every family member has those thoughts.

Your new life as a brain injury support person is similar to driving from New York City to Los Angeles. When you reach your destination, you will be given one million dollars. Oh, how you want to get there! You drive and drive and drive, never stopping for food or fuel. You are so desperate to get to Los Angeles all other thoughts and desires have been cast aside. Your life is being controlled by the need for a million dollars.

Time passes and you find yourself parked on the side of the road – still in New York – and out of fuel.

One of the reasons we are writing this book is to provide support for soldiers coming home from war zones with brain injuries. The War in Iraq, or any other war for that matter, consumes the news. The newspaper is filled with articles, magazines feature war photos on front covers, and television news reports story after story after story about the fighting. How much do you see about those soldiers in support units?

Those support units travel dangerous roads taking supplies to the front line troops. They take fuel, food, ammunition and much, much more to enable the "fighting" troops to persevere. Those pulling the trigger would not be able to do so for very long without the support troops doing their jobs.

When time comes to rotate the troops for much needed rest and relaxation, it's not just the fighting men and women who are rotated home.

Support personnel need rest and relaxation. They, too, need time away from the conflict, and so do you.

You find yourself becoming more irritated at little things. You become easily frustrated with your loved one; you want to scream, *"I've told you this a million times! Why can't you get it?"* You lie in bed at night, unable to sleep and unable to hold back the tears.

You are failing to provide what your loved one needs because nothing you do is working the way you had hoped and planned – at least that's the way it looks to you. You are rushing through the **Cycle of Response**, and there is not a "Stop" sign in sight.

People the world over have written many articles about how the human brain compares to a computer. If that were truly accurate, we would simply push the reset button – matter solved. But there is no reset button for the brain. Neither is there a magic pill that will make brain issues all better.

There is no reset button or magic pill to make your life as a family support member easier, either. You must recognize your limits. Pay attention to your fuel gauge. Know when that legendary straw is delicately poised over your back – the camel will need to take care of itself. It's your back that is in danger of breaking.

Take time for yourself. Family members need their own support group. It is necessary that someone be available to assume responsibilities for a day or a night. Practice your own troop rotation for the exact same reason the military does – rest.

There are support groups all over the world that can provide assistance for your mental state. Millions of family support members are an email away. Family support forums on the Internet are plentiful. You could consider yourself quite fortunate should you find a local group that has regular meetings. We believe one of the most important sections of this book and our website is *Sources of Information.*

Behavior Adjustment Plan

Planning to teach accepted behavior is not unlike planning a vacation, planning a wedding or planning for your retirement. Fortunately you already have the first two tools you need, and they are the same tools we recommended for the brain injured person: pencils and paper.

Keep things simple. While there may be numerous behavioral issues that need to be changed, don't try to change them all at once. Prioritize the most offensive or those that are extremely out of character for the brain injured person. You do not want to create a *mall effect* while trying to be of assistance.

Communicate with your loved one. Involve them in the discussions. Frequent communication that is open and honest will speed the process of building trust. Communication and trust, in turn, will add speed to the learning process.

Be certain that you speak clearly and slowly since their brain is almost certain to be processing information at a slower pace. Please remember that a brain injured person tends to take things literally.

If you say that you will do something in a couple of minutes, you have about two minutes to get with it. You do not have five or ten; you have two. How many times have you been in a store and heard an employee say, *"I'll be with you in a minute"*? Five, ten, fifteen minutes later you are still waiting.

You knew it would take longer than one minute and you expected to wait a short while. It irritated you, didn't it, when that minute became ten or fifteen? How irritated would you have been had you taken that person literally to mean sixty seconds?

Along this same line is using language that you do not really mean. *"Oh, I could just kill that man."* Perhaps you wake up to a severe storm with thunder and lightning filling the sky and you say something like, *"What a beautiful morning!"* Your loved one has a brain injury; the brain still functions. They will look at that morning sky and wonder why in the world you think it's beautiful outside.

Brain injuries affect different people in different ways. The ability to process information will vary from person to person. It could easily take a considerable amount of time for you to find out how new information is being processed by your loved one. Patience will have never been more virtuous in your life.

You will want to speak for your loved one. You will want to nod in agreement even though you don't have a clue what they're talking about. You may even want to correct their grammar as they speak. Be patient and do your absolute best not to do any of those things.

Good communication requires that your loved one understand what you are saying and that you understand what is being said to you. One item you will always want to communicate is praise.

Praise proper behavior. All people, not only those with brain injuries, like to be told they have done well. The happiest and most productive employees are those who receive *pats on the back*. The rest of the world could benefit by giving more praise; for you, it's essential.

Encourage independence by allowing your loved one to perform a task without your help. An opportunity to fail also provides an opportunity to succeed. Think back for a moment about that first meal Beth prepared: the bowl of green beans.

Was it a failure? Well, to the extent that it was to be a meal for three people, it fell short of providing enough food. She did, though, prepare those green beans with the proper seasoning, and they were fully cooked.

My failure was that I provided no list for her to use in order to complete her task. I should have given her a short list containing those three items, and she could have checked them off as she prepared them. At the time, of course, we did not know she had suffered a brain injury and had lost all peripheral vision.

Developing a behavior adjustment plan will go a long way in reaching and re-establishing a successful lifestyle. Write it down. Keep it simple. Communicate openly. Praise little successes.

Attitude Adjustments

Who doesn't need an attitude adjustment from time to time? Even though a brain injured person is not a lesser person, they tend to think of themselves in that way. After all, they cannot do some of the things they once did, and they tend to think about the past.

The past, as bad as it might have been, is not bad now. It was a time when names could be remembered. It was a time when words were easy to grasp. It was a time of friendship, fellowship and fun.

The importance now, however, is looking to the future. Don't look at how far a person has fallen since the brain injury. Concentrate on how far he or she can climb from where they now are.

Donna Jones has a story very similar to Beth's. Donna was in a car accident, then in a coma for 48 days. She, too, was told she would not be able to work again or participate in some of her favorite activities.

Donna wrote that in addition to not being able to hold down a full-time job, she was also told she wouldn't be able to learn anything new. Nor, she was told, would she be able to live in *mainstream society*.

Seven years after surviving the car accident, Donna is a brain injury survivor as well. She has a job; she has skied down her favorite Colorado mountain. You can learn more about Donna at our website. She, too, has written a book about her experience.

Remember Donna and how she was able to stand at the top of a mountain and let her body, soul and mind drink in the beauty that surrounded her.

Less than ten years after her brain injury, Beth was scuba-diving near the island of Curacao about fifteen miles from Argentina feeding sea turtles and sharks! There are many success stories, and you can be one more.

A brain injured person, at this moment in time, may think that the past is where all their fond memories will be. While that may prove to be true for some, a large majority of brain injury victims will have opportunities to stand on top of a mountain or swim beneath the waves of an ocean or ride a roller coaster.

Good behavior, good efforts and good attitudes should be rewarded. The reward should equal whatever was attained. Family members can help plan milestone rewards and final success rewards for the many areas of achievements.

It is important to be honest about the injury. No professional member of the medical community and no family member should ever paint an unrealistic picture of possible future achievements. The medical community certainly does a more than adequate job in that respect.

We have never met nor read about a brain injury victim who received false hopes from the medical community.

I'll say it again: it is important to be honest about the brain injury and its impact on your loved one. Things you should not say would include, *"You'll be okay. I bet you're back to work in no time." "Your memory will be back to normal before you know it."* While it is essential that we provide encouragement, we must avoid going over the top with over-encouragement!

One of the best attitude and behavior adjustment tools is for the brain injured person to assume more and more responsibility for daily living activities. We learned a long time ago that the *"go everywhere planner"* and its many *"memory lists"* are an essential part of recovery.

The next chapter, **Little Ol' List Maker, You**, has many sample lists mentioned throughout this book as well as several not mentioned thus far. Learn how these lists can benefit your life. Download full-sized copies from our website and print them for your personal use. Oh, personal use does not mean you can sell them!

Chapter Ten

Little Ol' List Maker You

Medical Index

Health Insurance Information

Medications

Medical History – Family History

Doctors Offices Index

Doctor's Offices Individual

Reasons I'm Going to the Doctor

How to Put On Makeup

Meal Planning and Meal Preparation

House Cleaning Checklist

Grocery List

Shopping List – Gift List

Travel Packing List

Travel Planner – Airline Strategies

What Do I Take When I Leave the House?

Work Strategies

Lists are an essential strategy that will help you in so many situations, from the doctor's office, to getting ready for work, to grocery shopping, to performing your job functions.

The next few pages contain sample lists that we used to help Beth resume activities with as little stress as possible. Please remember these are sample lists. Our actual lists contain brand names, size information, and other notes.

Each list is important; the medical lists are nothing short of essential. All of these lists are available in full page format on our website. They are there for you to download and use as a guide to make your own cheat sheets and *Memory Magic Planner*.

Each of these lists should be put in your planner. All you need is a three-ring binder that also has a place to put a letter-size pad of paper. You will need to take notes frequently, and having all your tools in one place will certainly make life easier and more productive.

Our goal is your goal: **Getting On With Life**. Keeping your planner up-to-date will help keep you on that path.

The Medical Cheat Sheet Index is simply a list of all the Medical Cheat Sheets in your planner. Write this list in the order the cheat sheets are placed in the planner to make it much simpler to find the information.

Medical Index	
List	Notes
Medications	
Health Insurance	
Medical History	Surgeries & Diseases
Family History	Diseases
Doctors Index	List of all doctors in my planner
Doctors Offices	Office information and driving directions

Think of your Medical Index as a guide to all your medical information. The next page in your planner will contain information about medications you are taking. The page after that will contain your Health Insurance information. Then your personal medical history will list any diseases and surgeries you have had such as measles, mumps, chicken pox, or appendectomy.

Medications Cheat Sheet

Medication Information	
Medications I'm Taking:	
Prescriptions:	
Migraines	Name of drug and amount in mg
Blood Pressure	Name of drug and amount in mg
Thyroid replacement	Name of drug and amount in mg
What I take it for	What it is
What I take it for	What it is
What I take it for	What it is
What I take it for	What it is
Over-the-Counter:	
Mild Aches	Ibuprofen
What I take it for	What it is
What I take it for	What it is
What I take it for	What it is
What I take it for	What it is
Notes	

Health Insurance Information Cheat Sheet

Health Insurance Information	
Health Insurance Company:	
Policy Number:	
Group Number:	
Member Name:	
Customer Service Phone:	
Primary Care Physician:	
PCP Address:	
PCP Phone:	
Supplemental Health Insurance Company:	
Policy Number:	
Group Number:	
Member Name:	
Customer Service Phone:	
Primary Care Physician:	
PCP Address:	
PCP Phone:	
Dental Insurance Company:	
Policy Number:	
Group Number:	
Member Name:	
Customer Service Phone:	
Primary Care Dentist:	
PCP Address:	
PCP Phone:	

Medical History

Medical History Information	
Chicken Pox	1981
Measles	1982
Mumps	Have not had
Broke Right Arm	1995
Tonsillectomy	1983
Appendectomy	Have not had
Hysterectomy	1990
Brain Injury	1990
Timber Ridge Facility	1991 - 1992
Thyroid Removed	1993

Family Medical History

Family History		
Father:		
Tuberculosis		1960
Cancer		1972
Hodgkin's Disease		1972
Leukemia		1972
Condition	When	
Condition	When	
Condition	When	
Mother:		
High Blood Pressure	Long as I can remember	
Condition	When	
Condition	When	
Condition	When	
Condition	When	
Condition	When	
Brothers/Sisters:		
Condition	When	
Condition	When	
Condition	When	
Condition	When	
Condition	When	
Condition	When	
Condition	When	
Condition	When	
Condition	When	

The purpose for an index of doctors you visit is to easily allow you to know if you have information in your planner about that particular doctor. A sample page would look like the one below.

Doctor's Offices Index

Doctor's Name	Specialty	Phone	Street Address
Tom Smith	Primary Care	555-1823	800 Marshall Street
	Dentist		
	Cardiologist		
	Gynecologist		
	Nephrologist		
	Neurologist		
	O. T.		
	Ophthalmologist		
	Pediatrician		
	Physical Therapist		

The following page in your planner would be office information and driving directions for the first doctor listed. You would add additional pages for each medical professional listed on the Doctor's Offices Index.

Dr. Tom Smith
Phone: 555-1823
Arkansas Children's Hospital
800 Marshall Street, Little Rock
Turn RIGHT on Brookswood Road and go to Hwy 67/167 Service Road
Turn Right on Service Road and go to on ramp
Turn LEFT at on ramp to enter Highway 67/167
Stay in LEFT LANE and go past where 67/167 merges with I-30
Move to RIGHT LANE and go 3 miles to I-630
Take Exit 139 B onto I-630 and go 1.8 miles
Take Exit 2 B to Martin Luther King, Jr. Drive and go .2 mile
Turn LEFT onto Martin Luther King, Jr. Drive and go .1 mile
Turn RIGHT onto Maryland Drive and go .1 mile
Notes: Parking lot is at the corner of Maryland and Martin Luther King Jr.

Listing the reasons you are going to the doctor will insure that you mention all your symptoms. A sample page would look like this:

Reason for Doctor Appointment

Doctor's Name	Appt Date	Appt Time	Phone	Have Referral if needed (√)
Smith	March-07	10:00	555-1234	None

Symptoms

My nose is runny. My head is achy. I have a temperature of 101. I'm having chills at different times during the day.

Go through the steps of putting on your makeup and write them down as you go. Then take that list and tape it to your bathroom mirror or dressing table mirror. Thereafter, you will have that list to refer to and it will cut down on the time spent trying to remember what step is next. Eventually, after you establish a routine, you may not need it any longer and can remove it. I kept mine in a drawer for a while until I felt comfortable that I could do without it. Your list will be longer or shorter, depending on how vain you are. - Beth

How to Put on My Makeup
Wash your face
Apply Toner
Apply Moisturizer
Apply Foundation
Apply Blush
Use Brow Brush
Highlight cheeks, forehead, chin
Apply Eye Shadow
Apply Eye Liner
Apply Mascara
Apply Lip Liner
Apply Lip Gloss

Meal Planning and Preparation Lists

Planning and preparing a meal is actually very good therapy for brain injured people. It allows them to make a significant contribution to their family. It allows them to exercise a degree of independence. It provides a re-learning opportunity and helps answer that question, "What Do I Do Today?"

Getting a meal planned and prepared involves the use of two lists: one for planning what food items will be prepared and another for preparing those items.

The reason is simple. We have already mentioned that Beth could not remember how to cook. Brain injury victim Courtney Larson said the whole arena of cooking was a new world as she began to recover. Cooking is **not** like *riding a bike*.

The Meal Planning List is used to list all the items to be prepared, the utensils needed for preparation and which pots, pans or other containers will be used. The list also contains the food items and condiments that will be part of the meal and information about any recipes that will be used. There is an area for notes where you can add a reminder to add items to the grocery list.

Meal Planning			
When planning your meal, list all the ingredients you will need as well as utensils and necessary pots, pans and/or bowls. It's a good idea to get them out in advance. Do you need microwave safe containers?			
Food Item	**Ingredients Needed**	**Utensils Needed**	**Pots, Pans, Bowls, etc.**
Green Beans	**1 can of green beans, salt, pepper, etc.**	microwave safe bowl	
Fried Chicken	Chicken pieces already cut, salt, pepper, flour, cooking oil	Tongs or large fork, paper towels	Large bowl, skillet, plate or platter
Add to grocery list: cut up chicken (breasts and legs)			
Recipes to be used: Aunt Sally's Southern Fried Chicken			

Meal Preparation				
Food Item	Where to Cook	Time to Cook	Time Began	Check When Completed
Green Beans	microwave	5 minutes on power level 50		
Chocolate Cake	oven	Bake 20 minutes at 350 degrees		
Notes:				

House Cleaning List

Cleaning the house is a big project and needs to be broken down into small segments. Think of how any successful group plans its strategies. There is a starting point and a definite goal to be achieved. Wise planners will establish milestones between the *start* and the *finish*.

A House Cleaning List allows you to establish the same type of milestone. Rather than *"achieve 30% increase in sales in New York City by September 23"*, yours might be *master bedroom cleaned in 25 minutes*.

House Cleaning List				
Room	**Task**	**Tools Needed**	**Time Allotted**	**Done**
Master bedroom	Make bed		5 minutes	√ when done
Master bedroom	Vacuum	Vacuum Cleaner	10 minutes	
Master bedroom	Dust furniture	Dust cloth & spray	10 minutes	
Kitchen	Wash Dishes	Dishwashing powder	Load, turn on dishwasher	
You get the idea.				

Grocery List

Item	Item	Item
Hot Cereal	**HOUSEHOLD:**	Soft Drinks, Diet
Cold Cereal	Air Freshener	Coffee, Decaf
SALAD:	A/C Filters	Coffee Filters. 10-cup
Lettuce	Batteries - AA	Coffee Singles
Tomato	Batteries - C	Coffee Creamer
Salad, Bag		Orange Juice
Salad		
Dressing	Room Deodorizer	Tomato Juice
Carrots	Light Bulbs	Lemon Juice
Mushrooms	Wasp Killer	Hot Sauce
Bell Pepper		
Onion	**LAUNDRY:**	**DESSERT:**
Broccoli	Bleach	Apples
Cauliflower	Stain Remover	Oranges
	Detergent	Banana
	Softener	Strawberries
		Whipped Cream
PERSONAL:		Ice Cream
Alcohol	**Detergnt/Cleaners:**	
Baby Oil	Bathroom Cleaner	**PAPER:**
Bandaids	Carpet Cleaner	Aluminum Foil
Deodorant	Stain Remover	Paper towels
Dental Floss	Drain Cleaner	Bowls
Hand Lotion	Glass Cleaner	Toilet tissue
Mascara	Disinfectant Spray	Clear Wrap
Mouthwash	Toilet Cleaner	Forks
Peroxide	Window Cleaner	Facial Tissue
Q-Tips	**Dish Detergent:**	Plates
	Dishwasher	
Razor Blades	Detergent	Sandwich Bags

Generic Shopping List

The purpose of a generic shopping list is to help you get organized for any shopping trip. This should be a full 8 ½ by 11 sheet of paper.

Shopping List		
Where am I going?	What am I going for?	Notes:
Yvonne & Tom's Fine Art & Pawn Shop	1. Big screen TV 2. Stereo system with surround sound 3. Size 10 combat boots 4. Minnesota Bob hat	Visa card Be sure to try the boots on
Tony's Service Station	Gas for car	Visa card
Driving Directions:		

Gift List

The Family Gift List will certainly make shopping easier for birthdays, holidays and other special times of the year.

For Christmas shopping you might want to add another column with the title of **Budget**. What gifts are available within your overall budget? Buyer's remorse in January is not something a brain injured person needs.

Family Gift List				
Name	Preferences	Store	Size	Age
Larry				
Beth				
Blake	Sports, games		6	6
Cooper				0
Notes:				

Travel Packing List

Circle **Yes** when the item is packed.

Travel Packing List	
Put a photocopy of passport in luggage	
Things to Take	**Packed Yet?**
Passports	Yes – No
Medicine	Yes – No
Clothes	Yes – No
Shoes	Yes – No
Makeup	Yes – No
Skin care – soap	Yes – No
Shampoo – Conditioner	Yes – No
Comb	Yes – No
Beach Towels	Yes – No
Sunglasses	Yes – No
Money	Yes – No
Sunscreen	Yes – No
Toothbrush – Toothpaste	Yes – No
Camera(s)	Yes – No
Bug Spray	Yes – No
Items for Carry-on:	

Airline Travel Planner – Strategies

Reduce airline travel stress with good planning. Do as much advance preparation as possible to reduce last minute surprises.

Airline Travel Planner	
Note: If you will need special passenger services, notify the airline well in advance of your travel so they will be able to accommodate you. Check your itinerary frequently for any changes to your flight schedule.	
Item	**Done**
Reservations Made	Yes – No
Special Needs Arranges	Yes – No
Current Passport	Yes – No
Cash and credit cards	Yes – No
Bags Packed	Yes – No
Bag identification tags	Yes -- No
Know check-in requirements	Yes – No
Know security requirements	Yes – No
Have gate finding maps & directions	Yes – No
Notes:	

What Do I Take When I Leave the House?

A list of what you need to have with you when leaving your house may seem to some to be overkill. It is certainly not overkill when you roll your cart up to the grocery clerk and have no way to pay!

It's not overkill when you drive ten miles to your office and discover your security badge is still at home. Nor is it overkill when you find yourself stranded on the highway with no way to phone for help.

Shortly after Beth had been discharged from the hospital, she had a blowout while driving during rush hour on the Interstate. After a cell phone call, our oldest son changed the tire and followed her to a tire center where she could get a replacement. *Note: Take cell phone.*

The list on the next page is a memory jogger list to provide suggestions as you make your own list. It is easy to assume that not everyone who needs a list goes to the same places. There are some common areas, though, like doctor's offices, stores, work, etc.

Earlier in the book we presented a question on the minds of most brain injury victims, *What do I do today?* How about making a new list of things to do?

What Do I Take When I Leave the House?	
Item	**Checkmark**
For Work:	
Purse with Money and Drivers License	
Organizer	
Badge	
Laptop	
Glasses	
Keys (Car & House)	
Sunglasses	
Lunch	
Cell Phone	
For Shopping:	
Purse with Money and Drivers License	
Grocery List, Gift List, Personal List, etc.	
Pen	
Organizer	
Glasses	
Keys (Car & House)	
Sunglasses	
Cell Phone	

(Continued on Next Page)

What Do I Take When I Leave the House?	
Item	**Checkmark**
For Pharmacy:	
Purse with Money and Drivers License	
Organizer	
Prescriptions or list of prescriptions to pick up	
Insurance Information – should be in organizer	
Glasses	
Keys (Car & House)	
Sunglasses	
Cell Phone	
For Doctor:	
Purse with Money and Drivers License	
Notes about reason for visit	
Prescriptions and Over the Counter Medications List	
Insurance Information – should be in organizer	
Organizer – make sure medical section is done	
Glasses	
Keys (Car & House)	
Sunglasses	
Cell Phone	

Work Strategies

A written *"work reminder list"* needs to be a part of the planner you will be taking to work.

Work Strategies
Arrive early and take a few minutes to plan the day!
Check voice mail.
Check email.
Plan the day's activities (include breaks and lunch).
Number the activities and organize them by importance.
Consider the time required for each activity and distinguish between "urgent" and "important".
Set a start and end time for each activity.
Split large projects into smaller pieces to keep from getting overwhelmed.
When trying to concentrate on a project, don't be afraid to say "no" to more incoming work. You can say, "Can I get back to you later on that?" Another thing you can do is let your phone ring so the caller can either leave you a message or send an email that you can address later when you have more time to concentrate.
Either end your day early enough to clear your desk and organize for the next day, or leave a few minutes late to do so. It will make a big difference the next day. Also, if in the middle of something complex and you are still fresh, it is better to stay late and finish it if that is possible. On the other hand, if things are not going well, leave on time and take a fresh look the next day.

Your Co–Worker List

A major problem facing those living with brain injury is remembering names of people. Returning to work can bring numerous opportunities for confusion, and that's why we believe you should have a cheat sheet for work that helps you remember names of both people in your office and those outside your office with whom you do business.

Very few job responsibilities can be accomplished without assistance from others. You should have a list in your planner that contains the names of people that will be assisting you. That list should contain the department where those people are located, their phone number and email address.

Perhaps most importantly your list should contain a note or two about why you interact with that person. You will certainly want to include the Human Resources Department or the name of the person responsible for your paycheck, payroll deductions, and health insurance information.

There are many ways you can use this list. Give it a different name and use it to remember other people.

Co-Worker List			
(include outside contacts)			
Co-Worker	Department	Contact Reason	e-mail or phone #
Dave	Sales	Contact for internal quotes	djones@mycompany.com
Mary	Accounting	Contact for questions about invoices	800-555-6702
Bobbie	HR	Payroll	
Bill Jones	ABC Supply	Office Supplies	800-555-9876
Notes:			

Chapter Eleven
Sources of Information

"Knowledge is power to a brain injured person."

"I Can't Remember Me"

"TBI Hell: A Traumatic Brain Injury Really Sucks"

"Traumatic Brain Injury Survival Guide"

"www.braininjuryguide.org"

"Knowledge is Power to a Brain Injured Person," is a deeply held belief of Beth's. Both this chapter and the next contain many sources that will assist brain injury victims and their families.

It should cause excitement to course through your veins to know that so many brain injured people have achieved so much in their new lives. There are many good books of hope, inspiration and information available to you. Some are presented here, but we encourage you to find up-to-date information on our website.

I Can't Remember Me is written by Judy Martin-Urban and her daughter, brain injury victim Courtney Larson. This personal story is about how Courtney's car accident changed the lives of so many people. Reading it caused us to realize that as bad as things were in our life after Beth's injury, other people experience far greater tragedies. Like Beth, Courtney's return to life after brain injury was one of returning to a new personality with new behaviors. She attributes *lists* as being a major help in her new lifestyle. More information about this book and family can be found on our website.

Brain injury victim George Gosling wrote *TBI HELL, A Traumatic Brain Injury Really Sucks.* If you are offended by salty language, this is not a book for you. It is written, remember, by a brain injured person. Written like a diary for the most part, the value of the book does not lie so much in what it says, but in how it is written.

It is a glimpse into how an injured brain works and, for that reason alone, we think you might find it beneficial. The book is published by Outskirts Press, Inc. and, of course, more information about it can be found on our website.

Dr. Glen Johnson is a Clinical Neuropsychologist who once was Clinical Director of the Neuro Recovery Head Injury Program. His *Traumatic Brain Injury Survival Guide* contains some of the most easily understood brain information to come out of the medical community. Find out more about Dr. Johnson and his book at our website.

Chapter Twelve

Professional Organizations

Brain Injury Associations by State

Selected Brain Injury Facilities

      Timber Ridge Ranch

      Methodist Rehabilitation Center

      Brookhaven Hospital

      HealthSouth

Note: Organizations listed here are for information purposes only and should not be construed as an endorsement by the author or the publisher.

State Listing of Brain Injury Associations

Brain Injury Association of America
Website: www.biausa.org

BIA of Arizona
777 E. Missouri Avenue, Suite 101
Phoenix, AZ 85014
Website: www.biaaz.org

BIA of Arkansas
PO Box 26236
Little Rock, AR 72221-6236
Web Site: http://www.brainassociation.org

BIA of Colorado
4200 West Conejos Place # 524
Denver, CO 80204
Website: www.biacolorado.org

BIA of Connecticut
333 East River Drive, Suite 106
East Hartford, CT 06108
Website: www.biact.org

BIA of Delaware
Brain Injury Association of Delaware, Inc.
32 West Loockerman Street, Suite 103
Dover, DE 19904
Website: www.biausa.org/Delaware/bia.htm

BIA of Florida
1621 Metropolitan Boulevard, Suite B
Tallahassee, FL 32308
Website: www.biaf.org

BIA of Hawaii
2201 Waimano Home Road, Hale E
Pearl City, HI 96782-1474
Website: www.biausa.org/Hawaii

BIA of Idaho
P.O Box 414
Boise, ID 83701-0414
E-mail: info@biaid.org
Website: www.biaid.org

BIA of Illinois
P.O. Box 64420
Chicago, IL 60664-0420
Website: www.biail.org

BIA of Indiana
9531 Valparaiso Court, Suite A
Indianapolis, IN 46268
Website: www.biausa.org/Indiana

BIA of Iowa
2101 Kimball Avenue LL7
Waterloo, IA 50702
Website : www.biaia.org

BIA of Kansas and Greater Kansas City
P.O. Box 413072
Kansas City, MO 64105
Website: www.biaks.org

BIA of Kentucky
7410 New LaGrange Rd. Suite 100
Louisville, KY 40222 **Website:** www.biak.us

BIA of Maine
325 Main Street
Waterville, ME 04901
Website: www.biame.org

BIA of Maryland
2200 Kernan Drive
Baltimore, MD 21207
Website: www.biamd.org

BIA of Massachusetts
30 Lyman St.
Westborough, MA 01581
Website: www.biama.org

BIA of Michigan
8619 W. Grand River, Suite I
Brighton, MI 48116-2334
Website: www.biami.org

BIA of Minnesota
34 13th Avenue NE, Suite B001
Minneapolis, MN 55413
Website: www.braininjurymn.org

BIA of Mississippi
P.O Box 55912
Jackson, MS 39296-5912
Website: www.members.aol.com/biaofms/index.htm

BIA of Missouri
10270 Page Ave, Suite 100
St. Louis, MO 63132
Website: www.biamo.org

BIA of Montana
1280 S. 3rd St. West, Suite 4
Missoula, MT 59801
Website: www.biamt.org

BIA of New Hampshire
109 North State Street, Ste 2
Concord, NH 03301
Website: www.bianh.org

BIA of New Jersey
1090 King George Post Rd., Suite 708
Edison, NJ 08837
Website: www.bianj.org

BIA of New Mexico
121 Cardenas NE
Albuquerque, NM 87108
Website: www.braininjurynm.org

BIA of New York
10 Colvin Avenue
Albany, NY 12206-1242
Website: www.bianys.org

BIA of North Carolina
PO Box 748
Raleigh, NC 27601
Website: www.bianc.net

BIA of Ohio
855 Grand View Avenue, suite 225
Columbus, OH 43215- 1123
Website: www.biaoh.org

BIA of Oklahoma
PO Box 88
Hillsdale, OK 73743-0088
Website: www.braininjuryoklahoma.org

BIA of Oregon
2145 NW Overton Street
Portland, OR 97210
Website: www.biaoregon.org

BIA of Pennsylvania
2400 Park Drive
Harrisburg, PA 17110
Website: www.biapa.org

BIA of Rhode Island
935 Park Avenue, Suite 8
Cranston, RI 02910-2743
Website: biaofri.org

BIA of South Carolina
920 St. Andrews Road
Columbia, SC 29210
Website: www.biausa.org/SC

BIA of Tennessee
151 Athens Way, Suite 100
Nashville, TN 37228
Website: www.biaoftn.org

BIA of Texas
316 W 12th Street, Suite 405
Austin, TX 78701
Website: www.biatx.org

BIA of Utah
1800 S West Temple, Suite 203
Salt Lake City, UT 84115
Website: www.biau.org

BIA of Vermont
P O Box 226
Shelburne, VT 05482
Website: www.biavt.org

BIA of Virginia
1506 Willow Lawn Drive, Suite 112
Richmond, VA 23230
Website: www.biav.net

BIA of Washington State
3516 S. 47th Street, Suite 100
Tacoma, WA 98409
Website: www.biawa.org

BIA of West Virginia
PO Box 574
Institute, WV 25112-0574
Website: www.biausa.org/WVirginia

BIA of Wisconsin
N 35 W21100 Capitol Drive, Suite 5
Pewaukee, WI 53072
Website: www.biaw.org

BIA of Wyoming
111 West 2nd Street, Suite 106
Casper, WY 82601
Website: www.biausa.org/Wyoming

Timber Ridge Ranch

Timber Ridge Ranch NeuroRestorative® Services, the facility where Beth lived for a portion of 1991 – 1992, is nestled on 315 acres of gentle rolling hills near Benton, about 40 miles from Little Rock.

"It may sound strange that I have many pleasant memories of living at a medical treatment facility. It sounds strange for me to say it. Turning off the rural highway to enter Timber Ridge brought a surprise. The facility actually looks like a ranch. It certainly didn't look like we were driving into a medical facility.

I remember standing in the library looking out the big window at the snow-covered fields and thinking how peaceful it was.

Both the Joint Commission on Accreditation of Healthcare Organizations (JCAHO) and the Commission on Accreditation of Rehabilitation Facilities (CARF) have accredited Timber Ridge.

What I remember most is the beautiful setting, a qualified and caring staff, a team that helps you establish and work toward goals, and how much they involved family members in the program. I was surrounded by others who were facing similar challenges to mine.".

Timber Ridge also has facilities at the University of Texas Health Center in Tyler, Texas, Hammond Place on the shore of Lake Ponchatrain in Hammond, Louisiana, and Oklahoma NeuroSpecialty in Tulsa, Oklahoma.

Methodist Rehabilitation Center

Accredited by the Commission on Accreditation of Rehabilitation Facilities and the Joint Commission on Accreditation of Healthcare Organizations, this facility is located in Jackson, Mississippi.

Learn more about this facility by visiting their website at www.methodistonline.org/ps_brain.htm.

Brookhaven Hospital

Brookhaven Hospital in Tulsa, Oklahoma is also accredited by the Joint Commission on Accreditation of Healthcare Organizations.

Learn more at www.brookhavenhospital.com

HealthSouth

HealthSouth facilities are located nationwide.

Alabama

HealthSouth Lakeshore Rehabilitation Hospital
3800 Ridgeway Drive
Birmingham, (205) 868-2000

HealthSouth Rehabilitation Hospital
1736 East Main St.
Dothan, (334) 712-6333

HealthSouth Rehabilitation Hospital of Gadsden
801 Goodyear Avenue
Gadsden, (256) 439-5000

HealthSouth Rehabilitation Hospital Of North Alabama
107 Governors Drive
Huntsville, (256) 535-2300

HealthSouth Rehabilitation Hospital Of Montgomery
4465 Narrow Lane Road
Montgomery, (334) 284-7700

Regional Rehabilitation Hospital
3715 Highway 280/431 North
Phenix City, (334) 732-2200

Arkansas

HealthSouth Rehabilitation Hospital
153 East Monte Painter Drive
Fayetteville, (479) 444-2200

HealthSouth Rehabilitation Hospital of Fort Smith
1401 South J St.
Fort Smith, (479) 785-3300

HealthSouth Rehabilitation Hospital of Jonesboro
1201 Fleming Ave.
Jonesboro, (870) 932-0440

St Vincent Rehabilitation Hospital
2201 Wildwood Ave.
Sherwood, (501) 834-1800

Arizona

HealthSouth Valley of The Sun Rehabilitation Hospital
13460 North 67th Ave.
Glendale, (623) 878-8800

HealthSouth Scottsdale Rehabilitation Hospital
9630 E. Shea Blvd.
Scottsdale, (480) 551-5400

HealthSouth Rehabilitation Institute of Tucson
2650 North Wyatt Drive
Tucson, (520) 325-1300

HealthSouth Rehabilitation Hospital of Southern Arizona
1921 West Hospital Drive
Tucson, (520) 742-2800

Yuma Rehabilitation Hospital
901 West 24th Street
Yuma, (928) 726-5000

California

HealthSouth Bakersfield Rehabilitation Hospital
5001 Commerce Drive
Bakersfield, (661) 323-5500

HealthSouth Tustin Rehabilitation Hospital
14851 Yorba Street
Tustin, (714) 832-9200

Colorado

HealthSouth Rehabilitation Hospital of Colorado Springs
325 Parkside Drive
Colorado Springs, (719) 630-8000

Florida

HealthSouth Rehabilitation Hospital of Spring Hill
12440 Cortez Blvd
Brooksville, (352) 592-4250

HealthSouth Rehabilitation Hospital
901 Clearwater Largo Road North
Largo, (727) 586-2999

HealthSouth Sea Pines Rehabilitation Hospital
101 East Florida Ave.
Melbourne, (321) 984-4600

HealthSouth Rehabilitation Hospital of Miami
20601 Old Cutler Road
Miami, (305) 251-3800

HealthSouth Emerald Coast Rehabilitation Hospital
1847 Florida Ave.
Panama City, (850) 914-8600

HealthSouth Rehabilitation Hospital of Sarasota
6400 Edgelake Drive
Sarasota, (941) 921-8600

HealthSouth Sunrise Rehabilitation Hospital
4399 Nob Hill Road
Sunrise, (954) 749-0300

HealthSouth Rehabilitation Hospital of Tallahassee
1675 Riggins Road
Tallahassee, (850) 656-4800

HealthSouth Treasure Coast Rehabilitation Hospital
1600 37th St.
Vero Beach, (772) 778-2100

Illinois

Van Matre HealthSouth Rehabilitation Hospital
950 South Mulford Road
Rockford, (815) 381-8500

Indiana

HealthSouth Deaconess Rehabilitation Hospital
4100 Covert Ave.
Evansville, (812) 476-9983

Kansas

Mid America Rehabilitation Hospital
5701 West 110th St.
Overland Park, (913) 491-2400

Kanasas Rehabilitation Hospital
1504 SW 8th Ave.
Topeka, (785) 235-6600

Wesley Rehabilitation Hospital
8338 West 13th St. N
Wichita, (316) 729-9999

Kentucky

HealthSouth Northern Kentucky Rehabilitation Hospital
201 Medical Village Drive
Edgewood, (859) 341-2044

HealthSouth Lakeview Rehabilitation Hospital of Central Kentucky
134 Heartland Drive
Elizabethtown, (270) 769-3100

www.braininjuryguide.org

Louisiana

HealthSouth Rehabilitation Hospital of Alexandria
104 North 3rd St.
Alexandria, (318) 449-1370

HealthSouth Rehabilitation Hospital of Baton Rouge
8595 United Plaza Blvd.
Baton Rouge, (225) 927-0567

Maryland

HealthSouth Chesapeake Rehabilitation Hospital
220 Tilghman Road
Salisbury, (410) 546-4600

Massachusetts

HealthSouth Rehabilitation Hospital of Western Massachusetts
14 Chestnut Place
Ludlow, (413) 589-7581

Fairlawn Rehabilitation Hospital
189 May St.
Worcester, (508) 791-6351

Maine

New England Rehabilitation Hospital of Portland
335 Brighton Ave. Unit 201
Portland, (207) 775-4000

Missouri

Howard A. Rusk Rehabilitation Center
315 Business Loop 70 West
Columbia, (573) 817-2703

The Rehabilitation Institute of St. Louis
4455 Duncan Ave.
St. Louis, (314) 658-3800

New Hampshire

HealthSouth Rehabilitation Hospital
254 Pleasant St.
Concord, (603) 226-9800

New Jersey

Rehabilitation Hospital of Tinton Falls
2 Centre Plaza
Tinton Falls, (732) 460-5320

HealthSouth Rehabilitation Hospital of New Jersey
14 Hospital Drive
Toms River, (732) 244-3100

New Mexico

HealthSouth Rehabilitation Hospital
7000 Jefferson St., NE
Albuquerque, (505) 344-9478

Nevada

HealthSouth Rehabilitation Hospital
10301 Jeffreys Street
Henderson, (702) 939-9400

HealthSouth Rehabilitation Hospital of Las Vegas
1250 South Valley View Blvd.
Las Vegas, (702) 877-8898

Pennsylvania

HealthSouth Rehabilitation Hospital of Altoona
2005 Valley View Blvd.
Altoona, (814) 944-3535

Geisinger HealthSouth Rehabilitation Hospital
2 Rehab Lane
Danville, (570) 271-6733

HealthSouth Rehabilitation Hospital of Erie
143 East Second St.
Erie, (814) 878-1200

HealthSouth Rehabilitation of Mechanicsburg
175 Lancaster Blvd.
Mechanicsburg, (717) 691-3700

HealthSouth Harmarville Rehabilitation Hospital
Guys Run Road
Pittsburgh, (412) 828-1300

HealthSouth Nittany Valley Rehabilitation Hospital
550 West College Ave.
Pleasant Gap, (814) 359-3421

HealthSouth Reading Rehabilitation Hospital
1623 Morgantown Road
Reading, (610) 796-6000

HealthSouth Hospitals of Pittsburgh
303 Camp Meeting Road
Sewickley, (412) 741-9500

HealthSouth Rehabilitation Hospital of York
1850 Normandie Drive
York, (717) 767-6941

Puerto Rico

HealthSouth Rehabilitation Hospital
Carretera #2, Kilometro 47.7
Manati, (787) 621-3800

HealthSouth Rehabilitation Hospital - Puerto Rico
University Hospital 3rd Floor Centro Medico
Rio Piedras, (787) 274-5100

South Carolina

AnMed Health Rehabilitation Hospital
1 Spring Back Way
Anderson, (864) 716-2600

HealthSouth Rehabilitation Hospital of Charleston
9181 Medcom St.
Charleston, (843) 820-7777

HealthSouth Rehabilitation Hospital
2935 Colonial Drive
Columbia, (803) 254-7777

HealthSouth Rehabilitation Hospital
900 East Cheves St.
Florence, (843) 679-9000

HealthSouth Rock Hill Rehabilitation Hospital
1795 Dr. Frank Gaston Blvd.
Rock Hill, (803) 326-3500

Tennessee

HealthSouth Chattanooga Rehabilitation Hospital
2412 McCallie Ave.
Chattanooga, (423) 698-0221

HealthSouth Rehabilitation Hospital
113 Cassell Drive
Kingsport, (423) 246-7240

HealthSouth Cane Creek Rehabilitation Hospital
180 Mount Pelia Road
Martin, (731) 587-4231

HealthSouth Rehabilitation Center
1282 Union Ave.
Memphis, (901) 722-2000

HealthSouth Rehabilitation Hospital-North
4100 Austin Peay Highway
Memphis, (901) 213-5400

Vanderbilt Stallworth Rehabilitation Hospital
2201 Children's Way
Nashville, (615) 320-7600

Texas

HealthSouth Rehabilitation Hospital of Arlington
3200 Matlock Road
Arlington, (817) 468-4000

HealthSouth Rehabilitation Hospital of Austin
1215 Red River St.
Austin, (512) 474-5700

HealthSouth Rehabilitation Hospital of Beaumont
3340 Plaza 10 Blvd.
Beaumont, (409) 835-0835

HealthSouth Rehabilitation Hospital of North Houston
18550 IH 45 South
Conroe, (281) 364-2000

HealthSouth Dallas Medical Center
2124 Research Row
Dallas, (214) 904-6100

HealthSouth Rehabilitation Hospital
1212 West Lancaster Ave.
Fort Worth, (817) 870-2336

HealthSouth City View Rehabilitation Hospital
6701 Oakmont Blvd.
Fort Worth, (817) 370-4700

HealthSouth Rehabilitation Hospital
19002 McKay Drive
Humble, (281) 446-6148

HealthSouth Rehabilitation Hospital of Midland/Odessa
1800 Heritage Blvd.
Midland, (432) 520-1600

HealthSouth Rehabilitation Hospital
515 North Adams, 3rd Floor
Odessa, (432) 550-1800

HealthSouth Plano Rehabilitation Hospital
2800 West 15th St.
Plano, (972) 612-9000

HealthSouth Rehabilitation Institute of San Antonio
9119 Cinnamon Hill
San Antonio, (210) 691-0737

HealthSouth Rehabilitation Hospital of Texarkana
515 West 12th St.
Texarkana, (903) 793-0088

Trinity Mother Frances Rehabilitation Hospital
3131 Troup Hwy.
Tyler, (903) 510-7000

Utah

HealthSouth Rehabilitation Hospital of Utah
8074 South 1300 East
Sandy, (801) 561-3400

Virginia

UVA-HealthSouth Rehabilitation Hospital
515 Ray C. Hunt Drive
Charlottesville, (434) 244-2000

HealthSouth Rehabilitation Hospital of Fredericksburg
300 Park Hill Drive
Fredericksburg, (540) 368-7300

HealthSouth Rehabilitation Hospital of Petersburg
95 Pinehill Blvd.
Petersburg, (804) 504-8100

HealthSouth Rehabilitation Hospital of Virginia
5700 Fitzhugh Ave.
Richmond, (804) 288-5700

West Virginia

HealthSouth Rehabilitation Hospital of Huntington
6900 West Country Club Drive
Huntington, (304) 733-1060

HealthSouth Mountain View Regional Rehabilitation Hospital
1160 Van Voorhis Road
Morgantown, (304) 598-1100

HealthSouth Western Hills Regional Rehabilitation Hospital
3 Western Hills Drive
Parkersburg, (304) 420-1300

A Special Thank You from Beth

My part of the book is dedicated to: Larry – who stood by me and loved me no matter what and who kept our family close together during this tragic time in our lives. Through our worst times, he continued to be there for our children while meeting his obligations at work and, yet, he was still always there for me when I needed him. He's the love of my life and my best friend.

Mom & Dad – who were there for me during the entire hospital stay and beyond. The last week I was in the hospital, I remember talking to my mom for what seemed like hours discussing what had happened to me and what was going on in the world. My Dad made sure I got the exercise I needed to regain my strength -- up and down the hospital hall, oxygen tank trailing behind.

My brother Phil, who was there for Mom, Dad and Larry, took on the responsibility of making sure the family had every last bit of the latest information about my condition. I'm told no nurse or doctor could escape without sharing all they knew.

My son Sean, who only 13 at the time, grew up to be a wonderful, successful young man. Although his mom did not die in the hospital, he went a long time without a mother even after I came home. Too many days I was in the bed with a migraine when he came home from school. I'm so thankful he made the right decisions during that critical part of his life when he had so many choices to make. His "Welcome Home Mom" sign I saw as we pulled into the driveway when I came home from the hospital is a sight I will never forget.

My son Chad, starting his second year of college and trying to deal with his mom being critically ill, was under such pressure for a young man just beginning a new chapter in his life. My worst day in the hospital was on his birthday. He handled the pressure of it all true to his personality and spirit. He even gave me a t-shirt after I got out of the hospital that said "JAMESON, takes a lickin but keeps on tickin." He always knew I would be okay.

My brother Ricky, who I remember holding my hand while in the hospital, talking to me with tears in his eyes. I was unable to communicate with him at the time, but I remember how comforting it was to know he cared so much.

And a special *thank you* to the team of medical and legal professionals who helped me achieve a successful lifestyle after my brain injury.

W. Kirk Riley, M.D, Primary Care Physician
Sidney Hayes, M.D., specialist
Jim Wellons, M. D., specialist
Robert Lehmberg, M.D., specialist
Ed Bethune, attorney
Laurence R. Dry, M.D., J.D., doctor and attorney
Mary L. Corbitt, M.D., headache specialist
Charles Wood, PhD, psychologist
Lisa Schlict, M.D., specialist
Dennis L. Wingfield, M.D., specialist
John E. Slayden, M.D., specialist
Tommie Flowers, L.C.S.W., A.C.S.W.
Ted Hood, M.D.
Patricia Debon, physical therapist
Sherri Eason, occupational therapist
Kellye James, speech pathologist
Barbara Bunten, social worker
Pat Raper, L.P.T.N.

The Beginning

You have reached the conclusion of this book, *Brain Injury Survivor's Guide*, and also the beginning of your new life as a Brain Injury Survivor family.

Welcome to Our World. It is a world of hope, and it is a world of frustration. It is a world of opportunities, and it is a world of confusion. It is the world in which we have lived for seventeen years and, now, it is your world.

We invite you to join with us at the website that is dedicated to providing you with even more information and an opportunity to interact with others in our world.

www.braininjuryguide.org

Welcome to Our World

LaVergne, TN USA
28 January 2010
171411LV00001B/41/A